New Methods of
Sensory Visual Testing

Michael Wall   Alfredo A. Sadun
Editors

New Methods of
Sensory Visual Testing

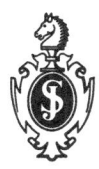

Springer-Verlag
New York Berlin Heidelberg
London Paris Tokyo Hong Kong

Michael Wall
Department of Psychiatry
and Neurology
Tulane University
School of Medicine
New Orleans, LA 70112, USA

Alfredo A. Sadun
Estelle Doheny Eye Institute
Los Angeles, CA 90033, USA

Library of Congress Cataloging-in-Publication Data

New methods of sensory visual testing / edited by Michael Wall,
   Alfredo A. Sadun.
      p.   cm.
   ISBN-13:978-1-4613-8837-1
   1. Neuroophthalmology. 2. Vision—Testing. I. Wall, Michael.
  II. Sadun, Alfredo A.
  RE725.N495 1989
  617.7'15—dc20   89-36801

Printed on acid-free paper.

© 1989 Springer-Verlag New York Inc.
Softcover reprint of the hardcover 1st edition 1989

Camera-ready copy prepared by the authors using Microsoft Word 4.0.

9 8 7 6 5 4 3 2 1

ISBN-13:978-1-4613-8837-1   e-ISBN-13:978-1-4613-8835-7
DOI: 10.1007/978-1-4613-8835-7

To our understanding and tolerant families,

Preface

Measurement of visual acuity has been the cornerstone of visual testing since Snellen began quantitating visual acuity using letter optotypes in the 1860s. Bjerrum in the 1880s brought sophistication and quantitation to the assessment of the visual field with tangent screen examination using differently sized and colored targets. Further advances in visual testing did not occur until the Goldmann perimeter and the Farnsworth Munsell 100 Hue test were introduced in the 1940s, permitting further refinement in the detection and quantitation of acquired visual loss.

An explosion of interest in sensory visual function testing followed the demonstration by Quigley and his colleagues in 1982 that despite the loss of more than 40% of the axons in the optic nerve, Snellen acuity and kinetic perimetry remained normal. Much of this interest has focused on a search for more sensitive and disease-specific sensory visual tests. Previously, novel tests used to probe visual function remained in the province of the visual physiologist and psychophysicist. These tests are now being introduced by the ophthalmologist into clinical practice. Concomitantly, the mass production of microcomputers and other technical advances have made tests such as automated perimetry and visual evoked response testing affordable for most offices.

The clinician is presently being inundated with a plethora of visual function tests that may require a knowledge of visual psychophysics and statistics to understand and interpret. The purpose of this book is to acquaint the clinician with these new tests so that they may be used to maximum benefit.

This book evolved from the 1987 symposium of the North American Neuro-ophthalmology Society on new methods of visual testing in neuro-ophthalmology. Dr. William Hart's excellent contribution on color vision testing has been published as a separate review of acquired dyschromatopsia in the Survey of Ophthalmology (1987). In lieu of a chapter on color vision, we refer you to this article.

We are grateful to our families for their forbearance. We are also indebted to our teachers who have inspired us to pursue investigations in sensory visual testing; they are, in alphabetical order, Drs. Ronald Burde, William Hart, and Simmons Lessell.

We also wish to thank our department chairmen, Drs. Delmar Caldwell and Stephen Ryan, for supporting and encouraging us to explore an area of medicine that requires a substantial investment in equipment, personnel, and time. Lastly, we wish to thank our staff and our patients for enduring the rigors of sensory visual testing.

Michael Wall
Alfredo A. Sadun

Foreword

This concise volume continues to prove that new techniques built upon existing information will transform ophthalmic science and practice during our professional lives. Thank goodness.

The previous generation, and in Neuro-ophthalmology that was the first generation, picked up whatever was at hand and used it to try to systematize how neurological disease affected visual function. Hand lights, direct ophthalmoscopes, tangent screens, and more than anything else the carefully taken history were put to use in the great detective task of diagnosis. Painstaking questions, exacting but inexact clinical examination, followed by the grand denouement, usually a craniotomy. It was the era of single case reports, sorted into bins to understand disease categories.

In 10 years, however, new imaging techniques have speeded up the process of correlation between clinical findings and those processes in Neuro-ophthalmology that are reducible to images in soft tissue. And, while new disorders still appear, the basic outline of clinical neuro-ophthalmology is set. The Holmesian methodology is still part of the fascination, but substantially more effort can be placed in using improved technology directed toward delineating the manner in which each disorder affects the visual system.

In order to do this, we must first understand the normal systems analysis of how we see. Chapter 1 by Carl Bassi in this volume alerts those who miss the basic literature in vision to fundamental change in the understanding of how our eyes process visual information. There is not simply one path for coded data from retina to visual cortex. Ganglion cells come in types with specific functional preferences. They are specialized in size, electrical responsiveness, and in their connections in the stages of the visual pathway. In parallel, different types of information is flowing together along the anterior pathway to be synthesized at the cortical level in our mammalian brains. It is well beyond the scope of this volume to review this material in detail, and the listed reference material is valuable for those who wish to know more. Nor can this book deal with other new findings that may provide substantial opportunity for new clinical testing. Rather, examples are provided to indicate that the bridge between the wet laboratory and the exam room can be productive and is a vital link.

We have all been aware for years of the importance of making a diagnosis with a tool that is uniquely designed to exploit the specific effect of the disease on normal function. Sex-linked red/green color blindness was studied intensively by psychophysicists at least in part due to its common occurrence in men. As the color confusions made by the affected eyes were understood, Ishihara and others had patterns painted that precisely isolated the "defective" perception from normal. From the point of view of the subject, the task is simple: a number either looks like a 5 or a 3. Children do it easily. The complex nature of the test is contained in the visual system of the subject, not in the difficulty of deciding what is seen, when it is seen, or in maintaining patience long enough to give a consistent answer. The pseudoisochromatic plate are so powerful a tool precisely because of elegant simplicity combined with the their targeting of the specific disorder's effects.

The aim of much of this book is to point to tests of visual function that may serve a similar role. Brightness sense, flicker, contrast sensitivity, threshold Amsler grid testing, and electrophysiological methods, as well as automated perimetry, deserve consideration as techniques that will aid us. It is, perhaps, too much to ask that every disease will have its own "Ishihara plate". But, we must not remain mired in the use of the same test for every disease where this clearly is insensitive. The performance of the same visual field study in a myriad of disorders of nerve cells each with a different effect makes little sense, except for initial screening. Even within the same disease, there are stages of damage that should be tested in different ways. For example, recent data on glaucoma strongly points to loss of one type of ganglion cell faster at the start of the process. Hence, in early glaucoma, tests should aim to isolate the functional loss associated with that cell type's favorite information. Eyes at a later stage of damage have little or no residual function of that type (the cells are dead), and different tests, for functions of the cells that remain, should be used. Thus, even within one disease entity, tests will ultimately be selected to maximize the available information.

The authors of this volume clearly understand and are working toward this ideal and we all benefit by their efforts.

Harry A. Quigley, M.D.
Professor of Ophthalmology
Wilmer Institute, Johns Hopkins University

Contents

Contributors

Carl J. Bassi, Ph.D.
Assistant Professor of Optometry
University of Missouri
St. Louis, Missouri 63121

Randall S. Brenton, M.D.
Department of Ophthalmology
University of Iowa Hospitals and Clinics
Iowa City, Iowa 52242

Karen Holopigian, Ph.D.
Postdoctoral Fellow
Department of Ophthalmology
New York University
New York, New York 10016

Mark J. Kupersmith, M.D.
Associate Professor of Neurology & Ophthalmology
New York University
New York Eye and Ear Infirmary
New York, New York 10016

Charles Maxner, M.D., F.R.C.P. (C)
Department of Ophthalmology
University of Iowa Hospitals and Clinics
Iowa City, Iowa 52242

Richard P. Mills, M.D.
Professor and Vice-Chairman
Department of Ophthalmology
University of Washington
Seattle, Washington 98195

Thomas E. Ogden, M.D., Ph.D.
Professor of Physiology & Biophysics
Department of Ophthalmology
University of Southern California/Doheny Eye Institute
Los Angeles, California 90033

Harry A. Quigley, M.D.
Professor of Ophthalmology
Wilmer Institute, Johns Hopkins Univeristy
Baltimore, Maryland 21205

Alfredo A. Sadun, M.D., Ph.D.
Associate Professor of Ophthalmology & Neurosurgery
University of Southern California/Doheny Eye Institute
Los Angeles, California 90033

William H. Seiple, Ph.D.
Research Associate Professor
Department of Ophthalmology
New York University
New York, New York 10016

H. Stanley Thompson, M.D.
Professor of Neuro-Ophthalmology
Department of Ophthalmology
University of Iowa Hospitals and Clinics
Iowa City, Iowa 52242

Michael Wall, M.D.
Associate Professor of Neurology,
Neurosurgery & Ophthalmology
Tulane University Medical Center
New Orleans, Louisiana 70112

Chapter 1

Parallel Processing in the Human Visual System

Carl J. Bassi

Introduction

Parallel visual pathways subserving separate visual functions have been well documented in animals. Evidence of similar parallel pathways have also been demonstrated in humans. This review is not intended to be a comprehensive overview of parallel processing; a number of such reviews exist (Rowe and Stone, 1977; Lennie, 1980; Stone, 1983; Kaas, 1986; Shapley and Perry, 1986; DeYoe and Van Essen, 1988). This chapter is meant to provide the reader with a general background of the evidence for parallel processing in the primate visual system, to extend that evidence to the human visual system, and finally to speculate that selective components of these parallel pathways may be compromised in certain disease states. This review also serves to make the reader aware of the many classification schemes used in describing parallel pathways and of the tests that may be used to assess the functioning of these pathways.

Evidence for Parallel Processing in Animals

The literature on parallel processing can loosely be divided into the pre- and post-1966 eras. Before 1966 the classification schemes for retinal physiologists were based on two major features of the ganglion cell output: receptive field characteristics and conduction velocity groupings in the optic nerve.

Hartline (1938) was the first to report that ganglion cells respond differently to light. "It is not until the bundles have been dissected down until one, or only a few fibres remain active that a new and striking property of the vertebrate response is revealed. For such experiments show conclusively that not all of the optic nerve fibres give the same kind of response to light." Some ganglion cells responded by increasing their firing and were teamed "ON" cells; others responded by decreasing their firing and were called "OFF" cells.

From this early description of ganglion cell types has come a number of classification schemes: X-Y; sustained-transient; pattern and movement; X-like, Y-like; alpha-beta; A-B; midget-parasol; magno-parvo; and M-P. Various anatomical, physiological, and behavioral evidence demonstrate the existence of parallel visual pathways subserving different functions in cats and primates (reviews, Lennie, 1980; Stone, 1983; Shapley and Perry, 1986; Lehmkuhle, 1985; Livingstone and Hubel, 1987). In the cat, Enroth-Cugell and Robson (1966) described two types of ganglion cells: X and Y cells. X cells are characterized by relatively small receptive fields, slower axon conduction velocity, and linear spatial summation; Y cells are characterized by larger receptive fields, faster axon conduction, and nonlinear subunit input (see Shapley and Perry, 1986).   These physiologically classified X and Y cells have morphological counterparts: beta and alpha cells. Beta cells are characterized by smaller dendritic fields and axons that project to layers A and A1 of the lateral geniculate nucleus (LGN). Alpha cells have larger dendritic fields that project to layers A, A1, and C of the LGN and superior colliculus. There is also a third type of ganglion cell: W cells that do not fit into the X or Y categories.

Similar evidence for parallel visual pathways exist in primates. Morphologically different classes of ganglion cells A and B (Leventhal et al, 1981) project to two different divisions of the LGN: the magnocellular and parvocellular layers. This segregation remains in cortex: the magnocellular layer projects to 4C alpha, which eventually projects to middle temporal cortical area MT (Zeki, 1969; Lund and Boothe, 1975). The parvocellular system projects to 4C beta, then layers 2 and 3 of area 17, to the "pale stripe" region of area 18, and finally to areas V3 and V4. As in the cat there are physiological differences between the systems. The parvo system is characterized by color-opponency, low contrast sensitivity, and high spatial resolution. The magno system is characterized by absence of color vision, high contrast sensitivity, low spatial resolution, fast temporal resolution, and sensitivity to stereoscopic depth. Figure 1.1 is a schematic of the proposed magno-parvo systems described in primates.

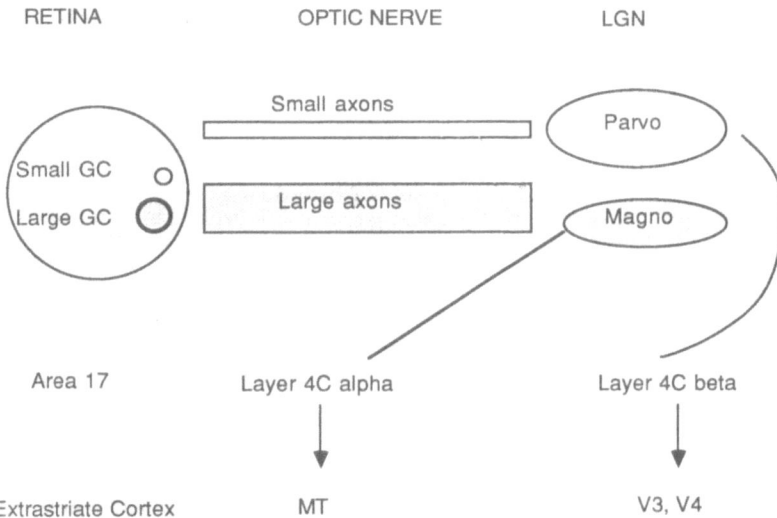

Figure 1.1. Proposed small cell/large-cell (parvo-magno) system in primates. GC = ganglion cell.

Evidence for parallel pathways have also been provided by toxin studies showing loss of different cell types in cats (Pasternak et al, 1985) and monkeys (Merigan and Eskin, 1986).

Evidence for Parallel Processing in Humans

Anatomy

Rodieck et al (1985) described different ganglion cell subtypes in Golgi-stained material. The two major types of ganglion cells were termed midget and parasol cells. These cell types likely correspond to the ganglion cell types A (parasol) and B (midget) characterized in primates (Leventhal et al 1981). Other ganglion cell types have also recently been characterized, e.g., "thorn" and "maze" cells (Rodieck et al, 1987).

A variety of anatomical and electrophysiological techniques have been used to demonstrate retinofugal pathways in animals. However, contemporary techniques for tracing axon pathways (such as tracer injections), immunohistological techniques, and the traditional method of utilizing silver-impregnation to follow degenerating fibers produced by an experimental lesion cannot be used in humans. Our understanding of the human visual pathways, until recently, was largely based on inferences from animal studies. Unfortunately, this indirect means of assessing the human visual system is inadequate, especially if one takes into account the interspecies variations documented in the experimental animal literature.

By means of the paraphenylenediamine (PPD) method, direct retinofugal projections to the LGN and pretectum have been demonstrated. The projections to the LGN were found predominantly in the lamina corresponding to the lesioned retinofugal pathway (layers 2, 3, and 5-ipsilateral eye; layers 1,4, and 6-contralateral eye). Transsynaptic atrophy was also noted among LGN neurons when the optic nerve damage existed more than two years. However, transsynaptic degeneration of either LGN neuron or the optic radiations was not found (Sadun, 1986).

This method also provided evidence for a direct retinofugal pathway to the pretectum. The fibers were found to originate from the most medial and ventral portions of the optic tract. The retino-pretectal fibers bypass the LGN and descend toward the pretectum via the brachium of the superior colliculus (SC) (Sadun, 1986).

The brachium of the SC was found to also carry retinofugal fibers that projected to the SC and to the pulvinar. The projection to the SC consisted of two parts: a large projection found in the deeper layers of the SC and a small projection to a superficial reticular layer that was organized in dominance columns separated by approximately 200μm (Sadun, et al, 1986b). A retinofugal projection was also noted to the pulvinar, with the concentration of degenerated axons being greatest in the rostral and lateral areas. As with the SC, the degeneration appeared to be greater in the pulvinar contralateral to the uniocular lesion (Sadun et al, 1986).

Retinofugal fibers were also found projecting into the human accessory optic system. The lateral, dorsal, and medial terminal accessory optic nuclei and the interstitial nucleus of the SC all showed degeneration following retinal or optic nerve lesions (Fredricks et al, 1988).

Finally, retinofugal projections were found in three areas of the hypothalamus. All three sets of retinofugal fibers were found to originate from areas near the optic chiasm: (1) Retinofugal projections were noted to both anterior and posterior lobes of the supraoptic nuclei. (2) Slightly more anteriorly, fibers from the retina were seen to course into the suprachiasmatic nucleus of the hypothalamus. (3) A fasciculus of retinofugal fibers left the most posterior areas of the optic chiasm, traveled between the two lobes of the supraoptic nucleus, and terminated in the paraventricular nucleus of the hypothalamus (Sadun et al, 1986).

Thus, eight primary pathways originating from the human retina and projecting to different areas of the human brain have been described. This suggests that different visual functions are being mediated at different anatomical sites.

Electrophysiology

Electrophysiological evidence for human parallel processing has been proposed by a number of investigators. Weinstien et al (1971) recorded extracellularly from individual human ganglion cells. They found evidence for different physiological types, including ON and OFF cells.

Evidence for parallel pathways has also been implied from recording visual evoked potentials (VEPs). Earlier evidence for parallel processing was implied from the finding that the latency of the pattern VEP to high spatial frequencies was longer than for lower spatial frequencies (see, e.g., Parker and Salzen, 1977). This finding was consistent with the findings that "Y cells" (i.e., low spatial frequency sensitive) had faster axon conduction than X cells. These findings, however, do not prove the existence of parallel processing. Other electrophysiological evidence for parallel processing has come from experiments measuring VEP amplitude at different contrasts (Nakayama and Mackeben, 1982; Parker et al, 1982; Murray and Kulikowski, 1983). These experiments have found a linear relationship between VEP amplitude and up to 10% contrast; at contrasts greater than 10%, the VEP amplitude increases much more rapidly (referred to as a higher gain in electronic terminology). These apparent different mechanisms acting at lower (less than 10%) and higher (greater than 10%) contrasts have been termed a "two-branched function."

In monkey, Nakayama and Mackeben (1982) found a two-branched function in the relationship between VEP amplitude and contrast. The gain (i.e., amplitude of VEP per unit contrast) of the VEP increases greatly at contrasts greater than 10%. This two-branched function (with a cutoff at around 10% contrast) was also found in single unit recordings from LGN cells by Kaplan and Shapley (1982). A similar two-branched function was found in humans by Parker et al (1982) and Murray and Kulikowski (1983). Murray and Kulikowski speculated that these two branches represented movement and pattern detection mechanisms. Previc (1987) proposed that frequency doubling of the pattern VEP occurs only under conditions that stimulate both the parvo- and magnocellular systems.

Psychophysics

Psychophysical evidence for parallel processing was discussed by Enoch (1978) in his quantitative layer-by-layer perimetry techniques. Enoch described two types of general responses, sustained-like and transient-like, that could be elicited by proper stimulation. These mechanisms were attributed to activity in separate retinal layers, with sustained-like function organized at the outer plexiform layer and transient-like functions organized at the inner plexiform layer.

Kulikowski and Tolhurst (1973) proposed two subsystems within the human visual system: movement and pattern channels. They found that near contrast threshold, a grating appeared only to flicker (the spatial structure was not seen) at low spatial and high temporal frequencies. At high spatial and low temporal frequencies the spatial structure was seen but the flicker was not. These systems have also been termed sustained-transient systems and have been related to the X and Y cells described in cats (the sustained system = pattern system/X cells; transient system = movement/flicker system/Y cells). This dichotomy of processing into separate channels has been challenged by a number of investigators including Lennie (1980) and Derrington and Henning (1981). Lennie (1980) found that X cells and Y cells do not form non-overlapping groups in spatial or temporal frequency sensitivity. Derrington and Henning (1981) established that the sustained system can transmit flicker information and the transient system can transmit pattern information.

More recent investigations have again found some evidence for separate mechanisms for visual processing (Martin and Lovegrove, 1987; Anderson and Burr, 1985; Pantle, 1983; Green, 1983). These investigators all tested sensitivity by either presenting stimuli on flickering backgrounds or with an adapting surrounding present. This factor may be important in distinguishing between the "parallel systems" in the visual system. These parallel systems might not carry distinct types of information but may be maximally (not solely) sensitive to specific stimuli. Thus, the pathways respond best to a type of stimulus yet still respond to all (or most) stimuli (also see DeYoe and Van Essen, 1988). Adaptation of one system by a stimulus more specific to one system can functionally isolate the other system. An analogous system is color vision. Different cone types respond best to a single wavelength, yet each cone type can respond to most wavelengths. By presenting a wavelength that adapts one cone type preferentially, one can begin to isolate processing in the other types.

Carney et al (1987) described evidence for parallel processing of motion and color information. Their conclusions are based on the findings that under specific conditions the visual system can exhibit binocular rivalry and integration of the two eyes.

Livingstone and Hubel (1987) provided a review of psychophysical evidence for parallel processing in humans. They further subdivide the primate visual system into three systems beyond the LGN: the magno system, the parvo-interblob system, and the blob system. These three systems have important differences in the type of visual information they convey. In LGN, a number of properties have been studied including color, contrast sensitivity, spatial resolution, and temporal properties. Whereas the magnocellular cells typically are not color-opponent, greater than 80% of the parvocellular cells do show opponency. Magnocellular cells are more sensitive to contrast and show a higher contrast gain (the change in response amplitude per unit contrast) than parvocellular cells. In addition, magnocellular cells have a lower spatial resolution and higher temporal resolution than parvocellular cells. In cortex, the parvo cellular and magnocellular systems further subdivide and three systems emerge. The magnocellular system appears to be most important for movement sensitivity and depth perception. It lacks color selectivity, has high contrast sensitivity, fast temporal resolution, and low spatial resolution. The parvo-interblob system appears to be important in fine detail discrimination, orientation discrimination, and shape discrimination. This system exhibits color selectivity, low contrast sensitivity, slow temporal resolution, and high spatial resolution. The parvo + magno-interblob system appears to be important for color perception. It is color selective, has high contrast sensitivity, slow temporal resolution, and low spatial resolution. Livingstone and Hubel (1987) presented evidence that corroborated previous studies in demonstrating that a number of properties important for movement perception and stereopsis were noncolor selective, had high contrast sensitivity, fast temporal sensitivity, and low spatial resolution.

Thus, there is anatomical and psychophysical evidence for parallel processing in humans. Might some diseases preferentially affect these separate channels?

Evidence for Parallel Processing in Disease

Glaucoma

In the primate model, Quigley et al (1987b) induced chronic experimental glaucoma in one eye in each of 10 monkeys. They found that there appeared to be a predilection for drop-out of larger optic nerve axons in the glaucoma eyes regardless of their position in the nerve. This finding supports the earlier description that there is a greater loss to the magnocellular layer of the LGN in glaucomatous-damaged eyes (Quigley and Hendrickson, 1984).

In humans, Quigley et al (1988) found that the smallest diameter optic nerve axons were preserved the longest in glaucoma. Consistent with this finding, a loss of larger diameter ganglion cells was observed in retinal whole mounts from patients with glaucoma (Quigley et al, 1987a). Figure 1.2 is a schematic of evidence for damage along the proposed magno-parvo pathways.

These anatomical findings have been followed up with electrophysiological and psychophysical findings. Trick (1985) reported that the pattern electroretinogram (ERG) was more attenuated for high temporal frequency stimulation in glaucoma patients. Both Tyler (1981) and Atkin et al (1979) demonstrated a loss of high temporal flicker sensitivity in patients with glaucoma. There is some debate as to contrast sensitivity losses in glaucoma. Ross et al (1985) reported losses in contrast sensitivity across all spatial frequencies in 60% of their patients whereas Adams et al (1987) reported no significant differences.

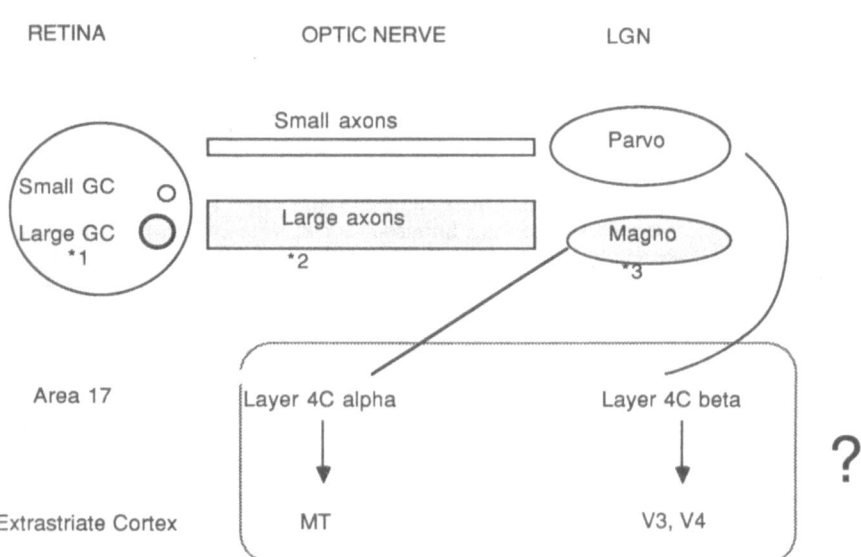

Figure 1.2. Evidence for damage to large-cell pathway: *1 Quigley et al (1987a) found damage to large retinal ganglion cells, *2 Quigley et al (1988) found damage to large optic nerve axons, *3 Quigley and Hendrickson (1984) demonstrated damage in the magnocellular layers of the LGN. ? = No evidence for specific cortical damage.

Amblyopia

Amblyopia, a functional visual loss that is not optically correctable, results from peripheral pathology. In animal models, lid-suturing one eye has resulted in severe amblyopia (which effectively eliminates pattern vision and attenuates retinal illumination in that eye). Lid-suturing results in severe anatomical, physiological, and behavioral deficits (von Noorden et al, 1970; Hubel et al, 1977; Blakemore et al, 1978; Harwerth et al, 1981; 1983).

In humans, amblyopia can develop from form deprivation that is less severe (e.g., anisometropia, unequal refraction between the two eyes, or strabismus). Anisometropia can be modeled in the primate using chronic atropine instillation in one eye. Atropine limits accommodation, thus causing an error in refractive balance between the two eyes. Kiorpes et al (1987), Hendrickson et al (1987), and Movshon et al (1987) showed that the long-term administration of atropine to the eyes of monkeys selectively compromised the parvocellular system. The monkeys demonstrated behavioral and physiological losses of high spatial frequency function, shrinking of cells in parvo layers of LGN, and diminished activity in layer 4C beta of visual cortex (Fig. 1.3). These results suggest that the small-cell pathway may be selectively compromised in anisometropic amblyopia (see also Sherman, 1979).

AMBLYOPIA

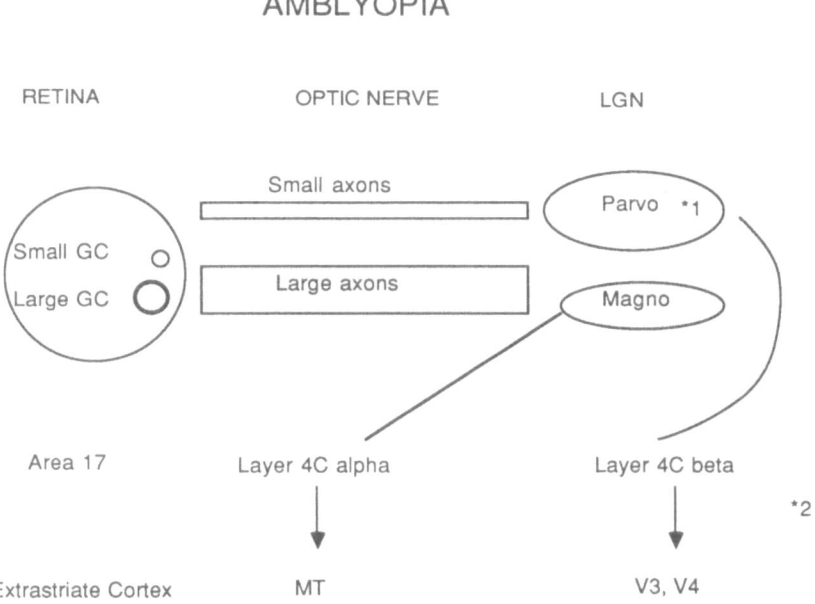

Figure 1.3. Evidence for damage to small-cell pathway in anisometropic amblyopia: *1,*2 Hendrickson et al (1987) found damage in the parvocellular layers of LGN and in layer 4C beta.

In humans, anisometropic amblyopia also typically impairs spatial sensitivity to higher spatial frequencies (Levi and Harwerth, 1977; Hess 1979; Bradley and Freeman, 1981).

A number of investigators have proposed differences in the underlying mechanisms of anisometropic amblyopia vs strabismic amblyopia. Under conditions of reduced illumination, strabismic amblyopic observers showed less detrimental effects on grating detection than anisometropic observers (Hess et al, 1980; Barbeito et al, 1987). There is also physiological evidence for differences between strabismic and anisometropic amblyopia in humans. Beneish et al (1988) found that the ratio of the amplitude of the flash VEP in the amblyopic eye to the nonamblyopic eye was significantly smaller between the anisometropic observers and controls but not between strabismic observers and controls, before any therapy. These findings support the hypothesis that there may be differential effects on parallel processing in the different forms of amblyopia.

Alzheimer's Disease

There is evidence that injury occurs in separate visual pathways in Alzheimer's disease (AD). Retinas from AD patients were compared with those obtained from age-matched controls. The retinas were evaluated through light microscopic examination of toluidine blue stained flat-mount preparations and also of PPD (Johnson and Sadun, 1988; Sadun et al, 1983) stained radial sections.

Whole-mount retinas were prepared and camera lucida drawings were made of all cells in the ganglion cell layer every 0.5 mm along the horizontal and vertical meridians and along the four meridians bisecting the angles between the horizontal and vertical planes. Cells were classified into definite ganglion cells, other neurons (likely smaller ganglion cells or displaced amacrine cells), and glial cells, based on staining characteristics. Comparable areas (at 5 and 11 mm from the optic disc defining mid and far periphery) examined in the retina of a patient with AD demonstrated a lower density of retinal ganglion cells. The drawings were traced on a graphics bit pad (MicroPlan II) system. Soma perimeters were calculated in more than 2000 cells in an AD patient and in an age-matched control patient. There was an overall loss of ganglion cells with perimeters larger than 40 μm in the AD retina (Bassi et al, 1987).

Examination of retinal PPD sections taken from AD patients revealed that certain retinal ganglion cells showed degenerative changes such as engorgement and microvacuolarization. These retinal ganglion cells also stained more darkly with PPD. The degenerating axon could be traced from the degenerating retinal ganglion cells to the nerve fiber layer of the retina. No degeneration was noted in the outer retinal layers. In addition to identifying degeneration in the retinas with whole mounts and with PPD staining of AD patients, examinations were also made of degenerated and intact axons remaining in the optic nerve (see also Hinton et al, 1986).

Fourteen optic nerves from 12 AD patients were compared histologically with 14 optic nerves from 12 age-matched control patients. The tissue was coded, and the amount of PPD staining was determined by a blinded observer. Significant degeneration was found in 10 optic nerves. These 10 optic nerves came from eight patients, all of whom had AD. However, four optic nerves from two AD patients did not have significant amounts of degeneration. All 14 nerves from the remaining intact age-matched control patients did not have significant amounts of degeneration.

The optic nerves from AD patients showed extensive degeneration as well as significant depletion of axons (a reduction, on average, of approximately 50% compared with the age-matched controls). These differences in the number of intact axons were reflected by decreases in axon densities in the affected optic nerves. The density of axons from the optic nerves obtained from age-matched controls averaged about 138 axons per 1,000 μm^2. This is slightly below the 150 axons per 1,000 μm^2 noted in much younger controls. However, the lowest densities of axons were found in patients in whom the presumptive diagnosis of AD was confirmed by the presence of plaques and tangles at autopsy. In this group the average axon density was only approximately 68.2 axons per 1,000 μm^2. Thus, the process of aging produced a small amount of axonal dropout whereas greater losses were observed in AD.

The cross-sectional area of the axons in the optic nerves, taken 7 mm anterior to the optic chiasm, was measured using an enhanced video-imaging system. There was a nonsignificant trend for nerves with a lower density of axons to have a greater mean diameter. This suggests the possibility that larger axons may initially be involved, with subsequent involvement of all axon sizes. In addition to loss of large axons, greater degeneration has been found in layers 1 and 2 of LGN from three patients with AD. Figure 1.4 is a schematic of damage to large-cell pathway.

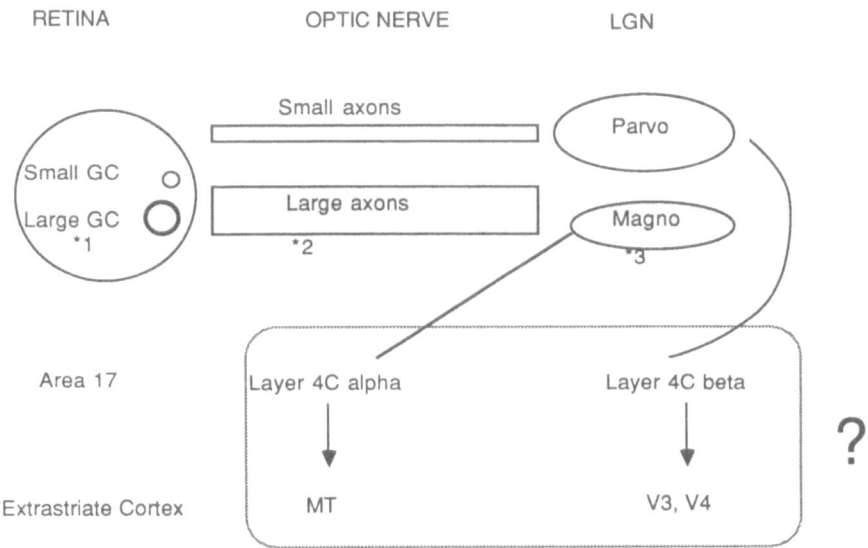

Figure 1.4. Evidence for damage to large-cell pathway in AD *1 Bassi et al (1987) found damage in large retinal ganglion cells, *2 Hinton et al (1986), Sadun and Bassi (1987) found evidence from damage in large optic nerve axons, *3 Sadun (1987) demonstrated damage to the magnocellular LGN ?=No evidence for specific cortical damage.

The significance of this preferential loss of retinal ganglion cell by size category is still subject to speculation. Thus, it is possible that in AD there is a predilection for degeneration of the larger cell pathway before a loss of the smaller cell pathway.

Fourteen patients with AD were given a battery of ophthalmological, neuro-ophthalmological, and psychophysical testing (see also Sadun et al, 1987). These patients were classified as having AD by established protocols of neurological, neuropsychological, and clinical laboratory tests. In general, certain patterns were noted in the clinical visual assessments of these patients. Patients who had relatively mild cognitive impairment would often complain of the inability to read. The AD patient, and more often his or her relatives, sometimes described "spatial" or "perceptual" problems. By this, the family usually meant that the AD patient misreached for objects on a table, thus knocking over instead of grasping objects.

Despite these complaints, mildly impaired patients invariably had normal Snellen visual acuity. Additionally, they usually had a normal general ophthalmological examination. In particular, their optic fundus appeared to be normal, and there was no evidence of optic disc pallor.

Nonetheless, even patients with mild AD displayed several abnormal features. The first common deficit was in the eye movement examination. The AD patients demonstrated long latencies in saccadic eye movements. The second common deficit was abnormal flash VEPs. Third, the pattern VEP latencies were sometimes delayed (130 ms) in comparison with the age-matched controls (about 110 ms).

The symptoms and signs in patients with moderate AD were often more severe. These patients had complaints similar to those with mild AD. However, their saccadic eye movements were even more delayed. Additionally, they showed dysmetria in both horizontal and vertical attempts at saccades. They were, however, able to maintain fixation fairly well. In patients with moderate AD, color vision was often impaired. Flash VEPs were often abnormal. The patients still had normal visual acuities by Snellen chart measurement and normal-appearing optic discs.

In severe AD, visual symptoms and signs were quite marked. These patients often had limited verbal capacities and said either nothing or simply that they "can't see." Because visual acuities were difficult to establish by Snellen chart measurement, we often had to use pediatric methods such as the "E game," Allen cards, picking up small white balls, or pattern VERs. Usually visual acuity was evaluated by at least two of these means, and typically the visual acuity would be in 20/100 to 20/400 range. These patients also demonstrated various degrees of dyschromatopsia. Mild amounts of optic disk atrophy were occasionally present.

In summary, 14 patients with AD were tested. Only one patient failed to show visual deficits. Most mildly impaired patients showed abnormal eye movements and VEPs while reporting "spatial" problems. Most had good visual acuities. More severely impaired AD patients often showed impaired eye movements, VEPs with poor visual acuity and color vision. Contrast sensitivity was measured in three patients using a Vistech chart. One subject with mild AD had a loss of contrast sensitivity at 6 cycles per degree (cpd); one moderate AD patient had loss of contrast sensitivity at 3 and 18 cpd; and one severely affected AD patient had loss in contrast sensitivity across all spatial frequencies. Many flash VEPs (five patients) showed a negative waveform flash characteristic of a very young infant's VEP. An ERG measured in one patient was normal but with an abnormal flash VEP; consistent with the anatomical findings of central pathway involvement with relative sparing of the outer retina.

These findings are especially intriguing in light of the findings of selective psychophysical functioning of parallel pathways in monkeys and humans. The preliminary anatomical results suggest that larger ganglion cells with larger axon diameters may initially be involved in AD. A great deal of evidence suggests that the parvocellular projection (or P cells) are involved in high spatial frequency and color discrimination. The magnocellular projections (or M cells) are important in movement, depth, and low contrast vision. This may explain the finding that ganglion cell loss may be found without loss of visual acuity.

Most provocative is the possibility that there is a predilection in early AD for loss of the largest retinal ganglion cells that are associated with the largest caliber axon fibers. Selective involvement of the large-cell system might explain the deficits in contrast sensitivity, spatial orientation, and eye movement control with only minimal effects on visual acuity.

Summary

In this chapter a variety of classification schemes for parallel visual pathways in animals and in humans are described. Perhaps the most difficult problem in reviewing the literature is the myriad of names used to describe the different systems. Most anatomical, electrophysiological, and psychophysical data support the notion that there are at least two systems involved in processing information (however, there is likely overlap in the information processing). There has also been accumulating evidence for a predilection for damage to one of these systems in some disease processes. Future research may find that careful testing of visual function may be helpful in the diagnosis of some diseases, in monitoring the stages of the disease process, and in evaluating treatment efficacy.

References

Adams AJ, Heron G, Husted R. Clinical measures of central vision function in glaucoma and ocular hypertension. Arch Ophthalmol 1987; 105:782-7.

Anderson S, Burr D. Spatial and temporal selectivity of the human motion detection system. Vis Res 1985; 25: 1147-54.

Atkin A, Bodis-Wollner I, Wolkstein M, Moss A, Podos SM. Abnormalities of contrast sensitivity in glaucoma. Am J Ophthalmol 1979; 88: 205-13.

Barbeito R, Bedell HE, Flom MC, Simpson TL. Effects of luminance on the visual acuity of strabismic and anisometropic amblyopes and optically blurred normals. Vis Res 1987;27:1543-9.

Bassi CJ, Blanks JC, Sadun AA, Johnson BM. The retinal ganglion cell layer in Alzheimer's disease. A whole mount study. Invest Ophthalmol Vis Sci 1987; 28 (Suppl): 109.

Beneish R, Lachapelle P, Polomeno RC, Lake W. VEP differences in strabismic and anisometropic amblyopia. Invest Ophthalmol Vis Sci 1988; 29 (Suppl):9.

Blakemore C, Carey LJ, Vital-Durand F. The physiological effects of monocular deprivation and their reversal in the monkey's visual cortex. J Physiol 1978;283:223-62.

Bradley AF, Freeman RD. Contrast sensitivity in anisometropic amblyopia. Invest Ophthalmol Vis Sci 1981;21:467-76.

Carney T, Shadlen M, Switkes E. Parallel processing of motion and colour information. Nature 1987; 328:647-9.

Derrington AM, Henning B. Pattern discrimination with flickering stimuli. Vis Res 1981; 21: 597-602.

DeYoe EA, Van Essen DC. Concurrent processing streams in monkey visual cortex. Trends Neurosci. 1988; 11:219-26.

Enoch J. Quantitative layer-by-layer perimetry. Invest Ophthalmol Vis Sci 1978; 17:208-57.

Enroth-Cugell C, Robson JG. The contrast sensitivity of retinal ganglion cells of the cat. J Physiol 1966; 378:379-84.

Fredericks CA, Giolli RA, Blanks RH, Sadun AA. The human accessory optic system. Brain Res 1988; 454:116-22.

Green M. Visual masking by flickering surrounds. Vis Res 1983; 23: 735-44.

Hartline HK. The response of single optic nerve fibers of the vertebrate eye to illumination of the retina. Am J Physiol 1938; 121: 400-15.

Harwerth RS, Crawford MLJ, Smith EL, Boltz RL. Behavioral studies of stimulus deprivation amblyopia in monkeys. Vis Res 1981;21:770-90.

Harwerth RS, Smith EL, Boltz RL, Crawford MLJ, von Noorden GK. Behavioral studies on the effect of abnormal early visual experience in monkeys: Spatial modulation sensitivity. Vis Res 1983; 23:1501-10.

Hendrickson AE, Movshon JA, Eggers HM, Gizzi MS, Boothe RG, Kiorpes L. Effects of early unilateral blur on Macaque visual system. II. Anatomical observations. J Neurosci 1987; 7:1327-39.

Hess RF. Contrast sensitivity assessment of functional amblyopia in humans. Trans Ophthalmol Soc UK 1979;99:391-7.

Hess RF, Campbell FW, Zimmern R. Differences in the neural basis of human amblyopias: the effect of mean luminance. Vis Res 1980;20:295-305.

Hinton DR, Sadun AA, Blanks JC, Miller CA. Optic nerve degeneration in Alzheimer's disease. Engl J Med 1986; 315:485-7.

Hubel DH, Wiesel TN, LeVay S. Plasticity of ocular dominance columns in monkey's striate cortex. Philos Trans R Soc Lond (Biol) 1977;278:377-409.

Johnson BM, Sadun AA. Ultrastructural and PPD studies of primate visual system: Degenerative remnants persist for longer than expected. Electron Micros Tech 1988; 8:179-83.

Kaas JH. The structural basis for information processing in the primate visual system. In Visual Neuroscience (Eds JD Pettigrew, KJ Sanderson, and WR Levick) New York: Cambridge University Press: 1986; 315-40.

Kaplan E, Shapley RM. X and Y cells in the lateral geniculate nucleus of macaque monkey. J Physiol 1982; 330: 125-43.

Kiorpes L, Boothe RG, Hendrickson AE, Movshon JA, Eggers HM, Gizzi MS. Effects of early unilateral blur on Macaque visual system. I. Behavioral observations J Neurosci 1987; 7: 1318-26.

Kulikowski JJ, Tolhurst DJ. Psychophysical evidence for sustained and transient detectors in human vision. J Physiol 1973; 232: 149-62.

Lehmkuhle S. Behavior correlates of physiological deficits in visually deprived cats, In R Aslin (ed) Advances in Neural and Behavioral Development. 1985; Vol 1, 107-29, Abex, NJ.

Lennie P. Parallel visual pathways: a review. Vis Res 1980; 20:561-94.

Leventhal AG, Rodieck RW, Dreher B. Retinal ganglion cells classes in the Old World monkey: Morphology and central projections. Science 1981; 213:1139-42.

Levi M, Harwerth RS. Spatio-temporal interactions in anisometropic and strabismic amblyopia. Invest Ophthalmol Vis Sci. 1977; 16:90-5.

Livingstone MS, Hubel DH. Psychophysical evidence for separate channels for the perception of form, color movement, and depth. J Neurosci 1987; 7:3416-68.

Lund JS, Boothe RG. Intralaminar connections and pyramidal neuron organization in the visual cortex, area 17, of the Macaque monkey. J Comp Neurol 1975; 159:305-34, .

Martin F, Lovegrove W. Flicker contrast sensitivity in normal and specifically disabled readers. Perception 1987; 16: 215-21.

Merigan WH, Eskin TA. Spatio-temporal vision of Macaques with severe loss of P retinal ganglion cells. Vis Res 1986; 26: 1751-61.

Movshon JA, Eggers HM, Gizzi MS, Hendrickson AE, Kiorpes L, Boothe RG. Effects of early unilateral blur on Macaque visual system. III. Physiological observations. J Neurosci 1987; 7: 1340-51.

Murray IJ, Kulikowski JJ. VEPs and Contrast. Vis Res 1983; 23:1741-3.

Nakayama K, Mackeben M. Steady state visual evoked potentials in the alert primate. Vis Res 1982; 22: 1261-71.

Pantle AJ. Temporal determinants of spatial sine-wave masking. Vis Res 1983; 23: 749-57.

Parker DM, Salzen EA. Latency changes in the human visual evoked response to sinusoidal gratings. Vis Res 1977; 17: 1201-4.

Parker DM, Salzen EA, Lishman JR. Visual evoked responses elicited by the onset and offset of sinusoidal gratings: latency, waveform, and topographic characteristics. Invest Ophthalmol Vis Sci 1982; 22: 675-80.

Pasternak T, Flood DG, Eskin TA, Merigan WH. Selective damage to large cells in the cat retinogeniculate pathway by 2,5-hexanedione. J Neurosci 1985; 5: 1641-52.

Previc FH. Origins, implications of frequency-doubling in the visual evoked potential. Am J Optom Physiol Opt 1987; 64:664-73.

Quigley H, Hendrickson A. Chronic experimental glaucoma in primates: Blood flow study with iodantipyrine and pattern of selective ganglion cell loss. ARVO Abstracts. Invest Ophthalmol Vis Sci 1984; 25(Suppl): 225.

Quigley HA, Dunkelberber GR, Green WR. Chronic human glaucoma causing selectively greater loss of large optic nerve fibers. Ophthalmology 1988; 95:357-63.

Quigley HA, Dunkelberger GR, L'Hernault NL, Baginski T. The sequence of retinal ganglion cell atrophy in human glaucoma: studies of optic nerve and retina. Invest Ophthalmol Vis Sci 1987a; 28(Suppl): 136.

Quigley HA, Sanchez RM, Dunkelberger GR, et al. Chronic glaucoma selectively damages large optic nerve fibers. Invest Ophthalmol Vis Sci 1987b; 28:913-20.

Rodieck RW, Binmoeller KF, Dineen J. Parasol and midget ganglion cells of the human retina. J Comp Neurol 1985; 233:115-32.

Rodieck RW, Dacy D, Watanabe M. Some other ganglion cell types of the primate retina. Invest Ophthalmol Vis Sci 1987; 28(Suppl): 261.

Ross JE, Bron AJ, Reeves BC, et al. Detection of optic nerve damage in ocular hypertension. Br J Ophthalmol 1985; 69:897-903.

Rowe MH, Stone J. Naming of neurons. Brain Behav Evol 1977; 14: 185-216

Sadun AA. Neuroanatomy of the human visual system: Part I. Retinal projections to the LGN and PT as demonstrated with a new stain. Neuro-Ophthalmology 1986; 6:353-61.

Sadun AA, Schaechter JD. Tracing axons in the human brain: A method utilizing TEM techniques. J Electron Microsc Tech 1985; 2: 175-86.

Sadun AA, Borchert M, DeVita E, Hinton DR, Bassi CJ. Assessment of visual impairment in patients with Alzheimer's disease. Am J Ophthalmol 1987; 104:113-20.

Sadun AA, Johnson BM, Schaechter JD. Neuroanatomy of the human visual system. Part III. Retinal projections to the hypothalamus. Neuroophthalmology 1986a; 6:371-9.

Sadun AA, Johnson BM, Smith LEH. Neuroanatomy of the human visual system. Part II. Retinal projections to the superior colliculus and pulvinar. Neuroophthalmology 1986b; 6:363-70.

Sadun AA, Smith LEH, Kenyon KR. Paraphenylenediamine: A new method for tracing human visual pathways. J Neuropathol Exp Neurol 1983; 42: 200-6.

Shapley R, Perry VH. Cat and monkey retinal ganglion cells and their visual functional roles. Trends Neurosci 1986; 9:229-35.

Sherman SM. Functional development of geniculocortical pathways in normal and amblyopic vision. Trans Ophthalmol Soc UK 1979; 99: 357-62.

Stone J. Parallel Processing in the Visual System. New York: Plenum Press: 1983.

Trick GL. Retinal potentials in patients with primary open-angle glaucoma: physiological evidence for temporal frequency tuning defects. Invest Ophthalmol Vis Sci 1985; 26:1750-9.

Tyler CW. Specific deficits of flicker sensitivity in glaucoma and ocular hypertension. Invest Ophthalmol Vis Sci 1981; 20:204-12.

von Noorden GK, Dowling JE, Ferguson DC. Experimental amblyopia in monkeys. I. Behavioral studies of stimulus deprivation amblyopia. Arch Ophthalmol 1970;84:206-14.

Weinstein GW, Hobson RR, Baker FH. Extracellular recordings from human retinal ganglion cells. Science 1971; 171: 1022-24.

Zeki SM. Representation of central visual fields in prestriate cortex of monkeys. Brain Res 1969; 14:271-91.

Chapter 2
Brightness Sense Testing

Alfredo A. Sadun

Introduction

Experimental animal and human studies have shown the existence of several retinal ganglion cell types, each with different central projections. These separate channels probably subserve different psychophysical functions. It is likely that several parallel visual systems exist in man and that each pathway subserves a different visual task.

There are many diseases that appear to selectively impair certain visual functions. For example, patients with optic neuritis often have good visual acuity but poor color vision. Quigley et al 1982 have shown us that patients with ocular hypertension (probably glaucoma) do very well in most routine ophthalmological screening tests, including color vision, visual fields, and visual acuity. Yet a postmortem histopathological exam of their optic nerves discloses severe axonal dropout. This reemphasizes the need to develop psychophysical tests that are more sensitive for the detection, characterization, and monitoring of visual dysfunctions.

Brightness sense determination has been described as "one of the most general rubrics in the psychophysics of vision" (Brown and Mueller, 1965). Hence, it has only recently been systematically tested and measured in patients with various disorders of the visual system.

Historical Background and Literature Review

Brightness Constancy

In a monochromatic setting a shade of gray is identified on a relative basis. Contrary to intuition, we do not describe an article as white simply because of the large amount of light that it reflects; nor do we describe an object as gray because of the moderate amount of light that it reflects; nor an object as black because of the minimal amount of light that it reflects. Rather, we take into account the general luminosity of objects seen in conjunction with the object of regard. Therefore, despite variations in general luminescence, a viewer will always describe objects that reflect the most light as white and those that reflect moderate or minimal amounts of light as gray or black by comparing each to the others.

Thus, it is not surprising that a white jacket seen in a typically illuminated office actually reflects considerably less light than a gray jacket would when worn outside in the bright sunshine. In the latter setting, the eye, recognizing the high intensity of luminous refractions of most objects in the sunlight, discounts the amount of light reflected off the gray jacket to a sufficient degree to lead to the visual impression of gray instead of white. The eye's sensitivity to light ranges over about 12 orders of magnitude. This enormous latitude almost mandates the need for relative measures of luminosity.

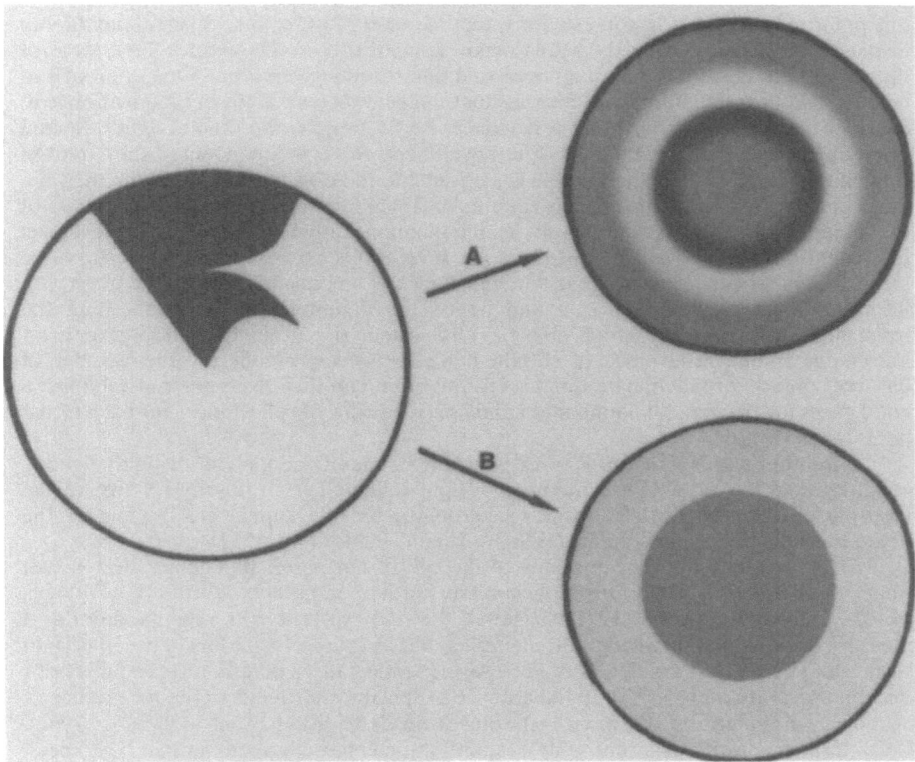

Figure 2.1. The Craik effect. Spinning of the Craik disc should produce the impression seen in "A" (above). The middle zone of "A" is a variable gray. However, the spinning Craik disc actually gives the appearance seen in "B" (above) of a homogenous light half about a homogenous dark half. Only the discontinuous point of the sector is appreciated.

The process by which comparisons are made in the assignment of various shades of gray is manifest in several optical illusions. One particularly revealing illusion involves the spinning disc that demonstrates the Craik effect. The Craik disc is colored white with a sector of black. If the disc is spun rapidly, most of it produces an even area of luminosity usually regarded as gray. However, as is noted in Figure 2.1, one edge of the gray sector has a discontinuity. This produces small incremental increases in the proportions of black to white as one moves centrifugally, except for one abrupt change. At this point there is a sudden jump toward a greater proportion of white, after which there is a gradual change back to the mean ratio. This leads to the outer third of the spinning disc having an identical mix of black and white as compared with the inner third. The middle third has varying ratios with an abrupt change exactly in the middle. However, the effect seen when the disc starts to spin is that the outer half of the spinning disc is perceived as light gray and the inner half as dark gray. The explanation is that the gradual changes in luminosity are not perceived; however, the abrupt change in the middle is. Since this abrupt change moving centrifugally goes from dark to light and all the other changes are gradual, the entire outer half of the disc is perceived as a lighter gray than the entire inner half.

Land and McCann (1971) in the retinex theory of color constancy, generalizes this point to establish a hypothesis for the perception of all colors. The retinex theory invokes a process by which the retina makes comparisons and integrates large areas of the visual field in establishing brightness and hue for any given area. One approach to help explain how the brain takes into account the general conditions of illumination is to consider the surface properties of reflectance. Reflectance is the ratio of light reflected by an object over the incident light. For most objects this is independent of the extent of total illumination. When illumination is restricted to the object of regard alone then the brain only has the numerator of this equation available to it; the perceived brightness of the object will depend entirely on its illumination rather than on its reflectance. However, in most physical settings there are several objects seen upon which the same incident light strikes. Knowledge of the reflectance of any object provides the brain with information on total illumination and hence the denominator for establishing the reflectance ratio for any other object. Less often, the brain does not have prior knowledge of the reflectance of certain items. However, usually a large number of different objects are illuminated and seen; the brain can take averages and establish a good guess for the general illumination and hence a series of reflectances for each of the items being regarded.

In other words, brightness sense constancy is maintained, under ordinary lighting conditions, as the ratio of the intensity of light reflected from objects relative to the intensity of light reflected from the background. Several animal studies suggest the ubiquitousness of this phenomena (Woodworth and Schlosberg, 1954).

As described above, the ability of the eye to normalize reflectance over a vast range of illumination leads to a phenomena termed brightness constancy (Wallach, 1948). Land and McCann (1971) suggested that the eye perceives brightness not as a measure of the total illumination on the retina, but as ratios of light flux between certain surfaces. These ratios are determined by surface reflectances that, in turn, require prior information (Kaufman, 1974). In the absence of specific knowledge of the reflectance of an object, a comparison between reflectances needs to occur (Von Helmholtz 1962). Cells termed "luxotonic," that only respond to changes in illumination have been identified by single-unit electrophysiology in monkey visual cortex (Kayama et al, 1979). Such a comparison could be due to different classes of retinal ganglion-cell-mediating responses to direct or ambient illumination (Richards, 1979). There is evidence of at least two classes of retinal ganglion cell responses in man. This has been demonstrated by several histopathological studies (Sadun et al, 1986a; 1986b) and by psychophysical studies (Enoch, 1978). Additionally, at least two types of retinal ganglion cell responses have been extracellularly recorded in human retina (Weinstein et al, 1971). These investigations suggest that parallel processing depends on at least two different response channels in the visual pathway. It is interesting to speculate that diseases may disproportionately affect these different channels, leading to selective impairments in brightness sense.

For all of its advantages, brightness sense constancy represents a loss of information by the visual system. Absolute intensity information is largely disregarded. Thus it appears that for survival value, information regarding relative intensities (reflectance) is more important than information about absolute intensities. The former is a manifestation of the property of objects themselves, the latter of ambient illumination (Cornsweet, 1970). What are the clinical manifestations of this relative nature of brightness sense?

Present Studies

Ophthalmologists are acutely aware that patients with retinal detachments frequently describe a dark shadow in the field corresponding to the detached portion of retina. Another familiar complaint to the ophthalmologist is the patient with anterior ischemic optic neuropathy who describes a dark curtain descending from above or ascending from below until it cuts his field in half along a horizontal line. Yet, the most common presentation of painless loss of vision to the ophthalmologist is probably that of the cataract patient who rarely describes a darkening of his environment (although he may complain of impaired contrast).

The neuro-ophthalmologist is familiar with the patient who has transient obscurations in vision due to disease in one optic nerve. Most commonly, the patient describes the entire visual field as becoming dark, sometimes to the point of complete blackness. A less common complaint is heard from patients with chronic impairment of one optic nerve who describe a diminution of brightness sense in the corresponding eye.

Patients with unilateral optic nerve disease most often will respond to direct questioning by describing the environment as appearing dimmer with the involved eye. They rarely complain that the entire room appears less than fully illuminated when looking through the impaired eye; rather, they describe specific objects as appearing less bright. For example, Goldmann perimetry often provides an opportunity for the patient to volunteer that the wattage for the illuminating light must be turned up or down, corresponding with the eye being tested.

Several neuro-ophthalmologists (Glaser, 1976) have described a diminution of color brightness with optic neuropathies. Mainster and Diekert (1980) described a simple device for quantitating color brightness.

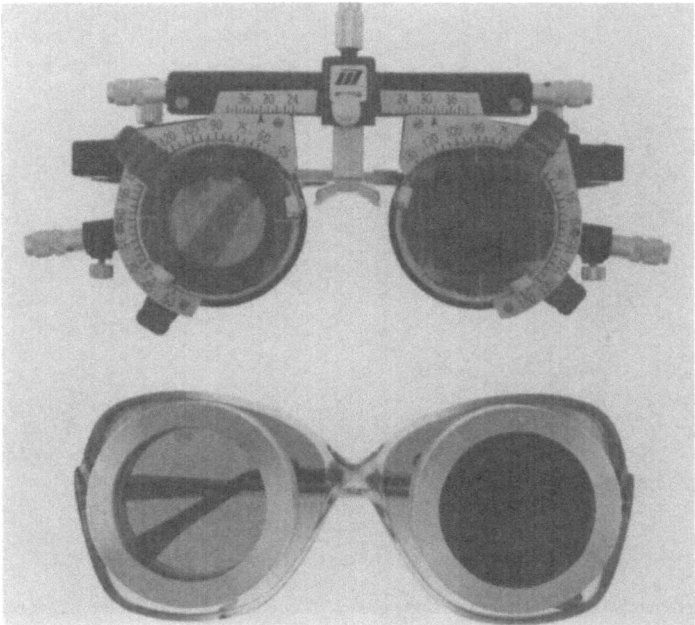

Figure 2.2a. Brightness sense glasses: two prototypes. Note that for each prototype the left ocular is set for maximum transmission; the right to limit light transmission.

These findings suggested to us that brightness sense is a function of the optic nerve that might be impaired by optic neuropathies. Therefore, the measurement of brightness could help in distinguishing and quantitatively monitoring optic nerve disease. We therefore developed a simple instrument for measuring brightness sense. Our experience with this instrument indicates that brightness sense can be used as a sensitive indicator of optic nerve disease.

Materials and Methods

The apparatus for testing brightness sense consists of a spectacle frame with a pair of polarized lenses affixed to each ocular (Fig. 2.2a). For each ocular the posterior polarized lens remains immobile; the anterior polarized lens rotates on a graduated carrier.

When the anterior lens is set at zero degrees, the two polarized lenses of that ocular have their gratings in parallel. This permits maximum light penetration (Fig.2.2b). When the anterior polarized lens is rotated to a 90 degree setting, the gratings of the two polarized filters are orthogonal, permitting minimal light transmission (Table 2.1). This device permits light transmission for each ocular to be varied continuously.

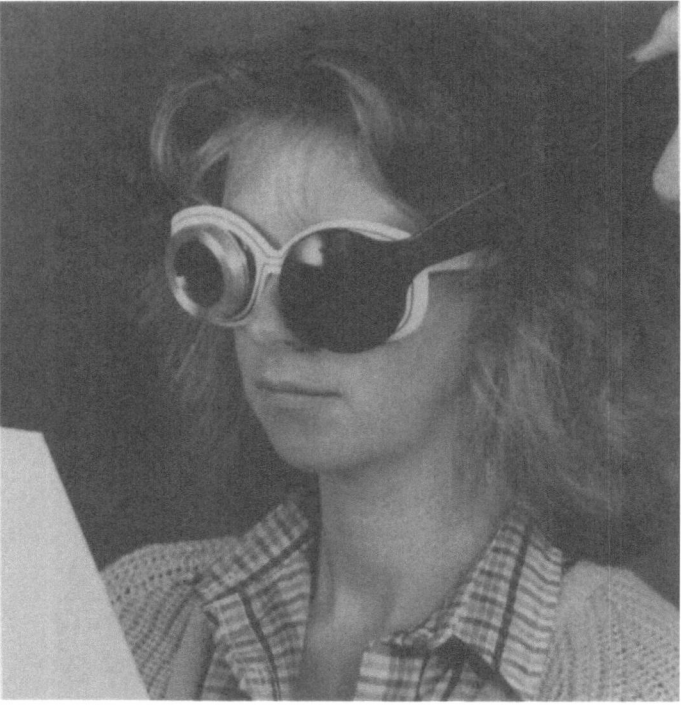

Figure 2.2b. Demonstration of brightness sense glasses. The subject or patient is looking at well-illuminated white paper and judging which eye sees it as brighter.

Table 2.1. Light transmission vs. the number of degrees
of rotation of the brightness sense glasses

Instrument Setting (deg)	Transmission
0	100
5	98
10	96
15	94
20	88
30	76
40	59
50	41
60	25
70	12
75	7
80	3
85	1
90	0

The observer wears the instrument as he would a normal pair of spectacles under standard room illumination. The observer is then asked to look at a sheet of white (nonglossy) paper, attending only to how bright this target looks and ignoring any issue of resolution or clarity. At the beginning of the test the anterior polarizers in front of both oculars are set at zero degrees. Each eye is then alternately occluded and the observer is asked to determine which eye sees the target as brighter white. The anterior polarized lens of the ocular through which the observer sees the target as brighter is then rotated to a higher setting. The procedure is repeated with each eye alternately occluded and the subject is asked to identify through which eye the target appears brighter. This process continues until the subject senses that the image is equally bright as seen through either eye. Sometimes the subject will describe the image as brighter in the eye that has not had rotation of the polarized lens. This requires "back titrating" of the polarized lens that had previously been moved. The process is continued until the patient sees the target as equally bright with both eyes. In other words, the polarized lens of the eye that sees the brighter target is rotated in order to neutralize the brightness disparity produced by an optic neuropathy.

The degree of rotation of this anterior polarized lens can then be used to calculate the amount of transmitted light through that ocular. The relationship between the angle of rotation and light transmission is described by the formula $I = I0 \times (\cos2 theta)$, where I indicates the light and I0 the illuminance. Table 2.1 demonstrates the amount of light transmitted at a variety of instrument settings.

Study 1

A total of 102 patients and twenty normal subjects were tested with the initial prototype brightness sense instrument. Most of the patients had unilateral optic neuropathies. The brightness sense values from these patients were compared with the brightness sense values obtained in several other visual disorders as well as in normal subjects. Additionally, impairments of brightness sense scores of all subjects and patients were compared with standard measures of decreased visual function including visual acuity, color vision, and afferent pupillary defects.

Study 2

We undertook this study with another 25 patients with optic neuropathies: 15 patients had anterior ischemic optic neuropathy and 10 had optic neuritis. All had monocular loss of vision. Static automated visual perimetry (Octopus) was performed to assess their visual field loss. Programs 32 and 34 were used; areas in which there was a loss of greater than 10 dB of retinal sensitivity were recorded.

Study 3

In order to study the relationship between brightness sense, visual acuity, optic disc changes, afferent pupillary defect, and color vision, we retrospectively analyzed another 300 patients in whom brightness testing had been done and selected 88 patients who had clear-cut diagnosed optic neuropathies. These optic neuropathies fell into the following categories: optic neuritis, n=47; anterior ischemic optic neuropathy (AION), n=23; optic nerve compressive lesions, n=8; other optic neuropathies, n=10. For all 88 patients one neuro-ophthalmologist conducted all measures of distant visual acuity, color sense, pupillary defect, optic disc appearance, and brightness sense. Visual acuity was assessed with the Snellen eye chart and the optimal refraction was used. Color vision was tested with either the Ishihara or A-O color plates. Correct identification of six or more plates out of eight was classified as normal. The pupillary examination was determined by the swinging flashlight test and classified on a 0 to 4+ scale. The optic disc was assessed by examination through a dilated pupil with both direct and indirect ophthalmoscope. It was classified as either normal, atrophic, edematous, or hyperemic. Brightness sense was measured using the device described previously in this chapter (Sadun and Lessell, 1985). Of the 88 patients who fulfilled the criteria described above, 41% were women, and the average age was 42 (range 9 to 82 years).

Statistical analyses were performed using analysis of variance to compare means across disease categories and also by Chi-square tests to compare the distribution of optic disc abnormalities across the disease categories (Sokal and Rohlf, 1981). The relationship between two measures of visual function were done by Spearman rank correlation coefficients (Sokal and Rohlf, 1981).

Results

Study 1

The brightness sense scores of patients with optic neuropathies were markedly different from those found in normal subjects (P < .001). Normal subjects were found to have a standard deviation of 9. We, therefore, arbitrarily defined a normal score as being greater than 82% of normal brightness sense (2 S D). Every patient with an optic neuropathy had brightness sense scores well below this cut off. Patients who had acute optic neuritis had brightness sense scores that varied from 2% to 40% of normal (mean 25%). Over time the brightness sense scores in patients with optic neuritis tended toward normalcy. After 3 months patients with unilateral optic neuritis had brightness sense scores between 25% and 75% (mean 45%).

Patients with ischemic or compressive optic neuropathies also had a significantly impaired brightness sense values in the involved eye (P< .001). For ischemic optic neuropathy the values ranged from 15% to 45% (mean 30%); for patients with compressive optic neuropathies, brightness sense values ranged from 1% to 35% of normal (mean 17%).

Patients with nonoptic nerve visual disorders sometimes had brightness sense diminutions as well. Patients with retinal disease particularly involving the macula showed modest diminutions of brightness sense (35% to 85%). However, these patients invariably had severe loss of visual acuity. In contradistinction, patients with optic nerve disease showed brightness sense impairments disproportionate to the severity of the visual acuity loss.

Patients with unilateral cataracts did not show diminution of brightness sense. This was true regardless of the severity of the cataract. One patient had a monocular cataract producing impairment of vision to 20/400, and yet she did not have decreased brightness sense in that eye.

Patients with factious visual loss were extraordinarily inconsistent in their responses even when each test was separated by only a few minutes. This is not surprising if one keeps in mind the visual system's capacity for a brightness constancy. In other words, there are no absolute values of brightness that can be recalled and matched by memory. The patient with factious brightness sense loss cannot reproduce the same level of gray that he artificially generated in previous tests.

In patients with optic neuropathies the brightness sense impairment was generally more severe than the effect on visual acuity. Brightness sense correlated best with dyschromatopsia and with an afferent pupillary defect. As the disease progressed, brightness sense was usually the first visual function to be impaired. Similarly, in partial resolution of an optic neuropathy, brightness sense was often the last function to demonstrate recovery. Visual acuity, color vision, visual fields, and even pupillary responses returned to normal by all conventional office testing methods in several patients with optic neuritis. Yet brightness sense remained impaired to approximately the 50% level; this corroborated the patient's description of a persistent subtle visual deficit.

Patients with organic disease that produced brightness sense diminution showed remarkable consistency on retesting. Similarly, all normal subjects gave consistent responses that almost invariably fell within 5 degrees of the initial settings. Patients with factitial loss were an exception as described above.

In review of these patients with optic nerve disease, several interesting patterns became evident. Patients with the diagnosis of optic neuritis frequently showed changes of brightness sense that preceded more profound changes in visual acuity and color vision. In general, the brightness sense most closely paralleled the afferent pupillary defect. During the resolution phase of the optic neuritis, brightness sense was also the first to improve; however, it rarely improved beyond 60% of normal. Brightness sense often remained the only clinical evidence of any optic nerve dysfunction several months after resolution of the optic neuritis.

In ischemic optic neuropathy the visual acuities would have varied considerably. However, three signs were consistently found: impairments in color vision, an afferent pupillary defect, and decreased brightness sense. Of these three, color vision was usually the least affected. We found the pattern of a marked afferent pupillary defect and profound loss of brightness sense in the presence of only mild impairment of color vision to be most characteristic for anterior ischemic optic neuropathy.

Patients who had cataracts or other media opacities did not manifest any change in brightness sense. Removal of the cataract produced an increased sense of brightness for hours after the cataract extraction. However, by two days at the most, brightness sense had returned to normal when compared with the fellow eye.

Study 2.

If brightness sense is mediated by a select class of retinal ganglion cells, then comparing the amount and areas of visual field loss with the brightness sense impairment might lead to appreciation of the distribution of the retinal ganglion cells that mediate brightness sense. (Figure 2.3a) demonstrates the relationship between visual field area loss centrally and brightness sense. (Figure 2.3b) demonstrates the relationship between general visual field loss and brightness sense. Several interesting observations can be made.

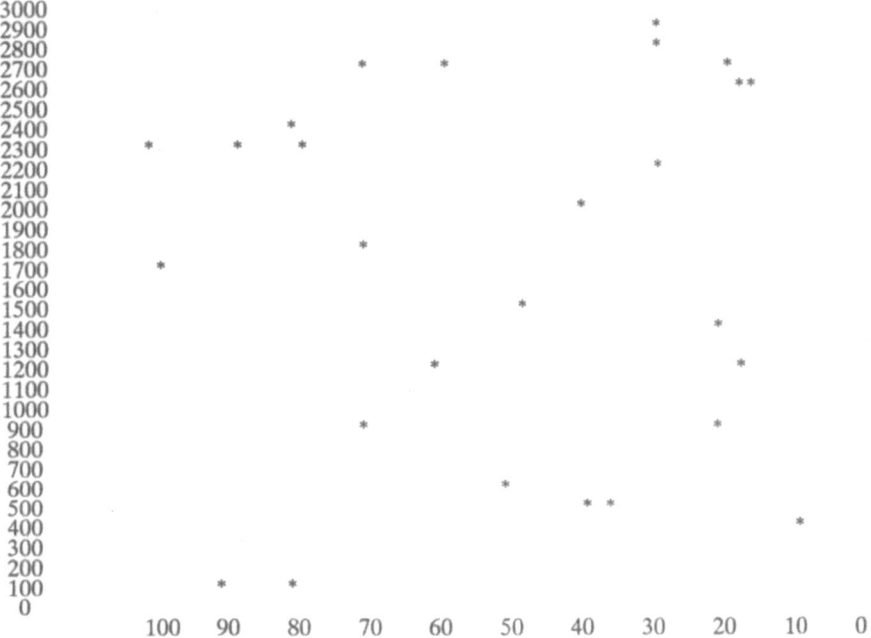

Figure 2.3a. Brightness sense vs. central field loss. There is no clear-cut relationship of brightness sense impairment (percent) to central field loss (in square degrees of area depressed 2 log units or more).

Brightness sense impairment did not correlate with central visual field loss in optic nerve disease! Most receptors and, indeed, most retinal ganglion cells are concerned with the central 10 degrees of vision. If all the retinal ganglion cells contributed equally to the sense of brightness, one would expect that central field loss would have a much greater impact on brightness sense than peripheral field loss. However, it has been observed clinically that patients often have losses in brightness sense that are out of proportion to losses in visual acuity. This suggests that brightness sense does not have to be largely mediated through the central field.

There was however, a striking correlation between brightness sense impairment and peripheral field loss. The correlation appeared to be linear for at least the first 70% of brightness sense loss and then became slightly exponential. Along the linear portion of the curve there was an approximate loss of 10% in brightness sense for every 1,000 square degrees of visual field loss.

Study 3

The percentages of eyes that had abnormalities for each of the visual functions described in each disease category are seen in Table 2.2. It can be noted that brightness sense was the most sensitive measure overall. It classified patients with optic neuritis, compressive diseases of the optic nerve, and other neuropathies as abnormal more than did any other measure alone. It detected 87%, 100%, and 80%, respectively, in these three disease groups. However, for patients with AION both pupillary defect and visual acuity were more sensitive measures for detecting abnormalities than was brightness sense. Only color vision testing was less sensitive as a measure for all disease groups, correctly identifying only 60% to 68% of patients in each of the four optic neuropathy groups as abnormal.   It is interesting to note that, particularly in AION color vision was considerably less sensitive in the identification of disease than any other measure.

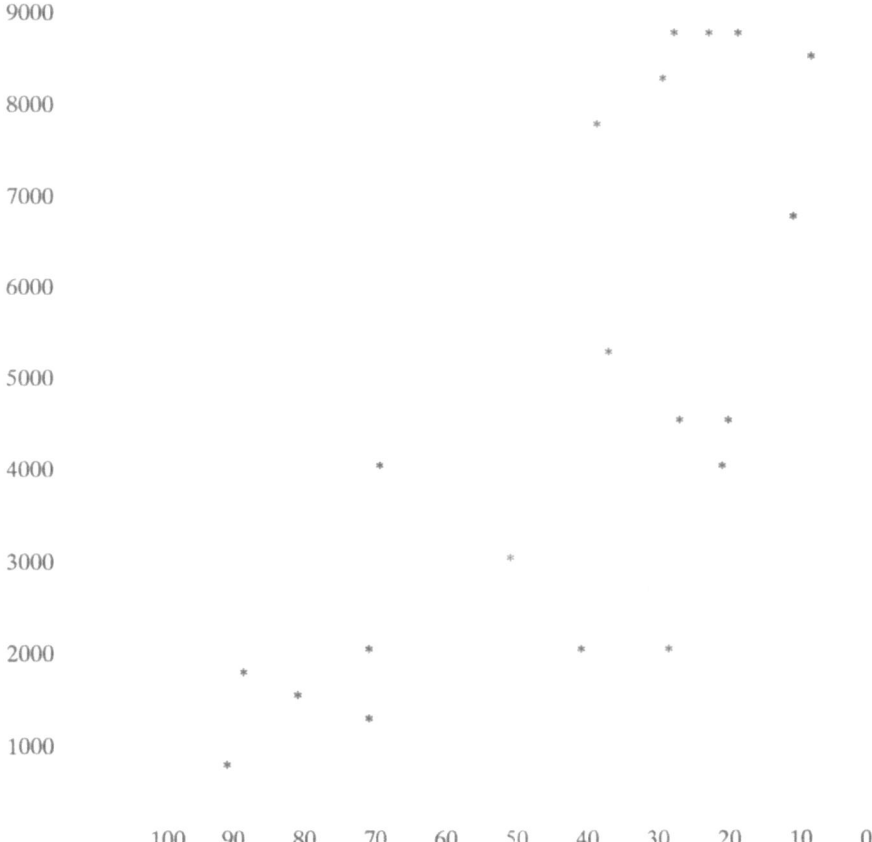

Figure 2.3b. Brightness sense vs. peripheral field loss. There is a near linear relationship between peripheral visual field loss (given in square degrees) and brightness sense impairment (percent).

The different mean values for brightness sense, pupillary defects, color vision defects, and optic disc deformities can be seen in Table 2.3. For the purposes of this table, pupillary defects were described as an afferent pupillary defect rated on a 1 to 4 scale; color vision defects were the number of plates incorrectly identified out of eight (A-O); optic disc defects were described as normal, atrophic, or edematous.In this table, only optic nerve head changes differed significantly between disease categories (P=.003). In other words, while Table 2.3 suggests that brightness sense is the most sensitive and reliable measure of optic nerve disease, Table 2.2 suggests that optic disc appearance is the most reliable indicator of what type of disease is impairing optic nerve function.

Table 2.2. Sensitivity of measures of visual function:
percentage correctly classified as abnormal

Test	ON	Comp. ON	AION	Other
Brightness sense	87.2	100.0	82.6	80.0
Visual acuity	76.6	87.5	91.3	70.0
Pupillary defect	74.5	75.0	95.6	60.0
Color plates	68.1	62.5	65.2	60.0
Optic disc	85.1	62.5	87.0	70.0

ON = optic neuritis, comp. ON = compressive optic neuropathy, AION = anterior ischemic optic neuropathy, other = other optic neuropathies.

Table 2.3. Mean values of visual function parameters and distribution of optic disc defects by disease category

Test	ON	Comp. ON	ION	Other
Brightness sense	42.0	33.0	42.4	57.5
Pupillary defect	1.3	1.3	1.6	0.6
Color vision	4.7	4.3	3.4	5.3
Optic disc defect				
Normal	15%	38%	13%	30%
Atrophic	45%	62%	74%	60%
Edema	40%	0%	13%	10%

ON = optic neuritis, comp. ON = compressive optic neuropathy, ION = ischemic optic neuropathy, other = other optic neuropathies.

Patients with acute optic neuritis often had edematous optic discs, whereas the remaining groups had optic discs that were likely to be atrophic. Brightness sense was significantly decreased from normal for every category of disease. Brightness sense, pupillary defects, and color vision test results did not show a statistically significant mean difference between disease groups.

Comparison between these four parameters of visual function yields interesting results: Spearman rank correlation coefficients were calculated. In optic neuritis brightness sense was significantly correlated with the degree of pupillary defect ($r = -0.47$), a decrease in color vision ($r = 0.43$), and a decline in visual acuity ($r = -0.47$). The magnitude of correlation of brightness sense with measures of visual function was lower in all disease categories except compressive disorders, where brightness sense and visual acuity remained moderately correlated.

Patients with AION demonstrated edematous discs and the greatest brightness sense deficit. Patients with AION who had atrophic discs showed less impairment of brightness sense. Patients with normal-appearing optic discs had the least impairment of brightness sense. Among patients with optic neuritis, edematous discs also showed the greatest brightness sense deficit, with atrophic discs showing only moderate impairment and normal-appearing discs demonstrating the least impairment.

Discussion

Visual acuity remains an important measure in the assessment of ophthalmic disease; however, it is evident that in many cases visual acuity alone is insufficient to detect visual deficits in general and optic nerve dysfunction in particular. The subclinical optic neuropathy prevalent among cases of multiple sclerosis and manifested only by losses in contrast sensitivity or visual evoked response abnormality adds further evidence of the inadequacy of visual acuity for the assessment of optic nerve function. Histopathological evidence from cases of glaucomatous optic atrophy further suggests that the threshold for detecting optic nerve lesions through routine office techniques is disturbingly high. Postmortem studies have shown that approximately half of the optic nerve axons had been lost in patients who had normal eye examinations (Quigley et al, 1982).

Brightness sense testing provides a new dimension in the evaluation of optic nerve function. Space does not permit a complete psychophysical analysis of brightness sense; however, it is clear that the sense of brightness is, as previously discussed, much more than a simple function of the total light flux that reaches the retina. The ability of the eye to normalize the gray scale over a vast range of illumination is termed "brightness constancy" and explains why a gray object may appear approximately the same shade of gray under vastly different illuminations (Wallach, 1948). The eye perceives brightness as ratios of light flux from various surfaces determined by surface characteristics and reflectances (Land and McCann, 1971; Kaufman, 1974). Thus, different areas of the retina, or perhaps different classes of retinal ganglion cells, must be compared for the determination of true surface reflectances (Von Helmholtz, 1962; Richards, 1979). Indeed, there is considerable evidence for the existence of different retinal ganglion cell types in the human retina (Enoch, 1978; Weinstein et al, 1971; Sadun et al, 1986a; 1986b; Rowe and Stone, 1977; Berson, 1981; Rodieck, 1979; Sadun and Schaechter, 1983). Certain types of injuries to the optic nerve might selectively damage the projection of only one class of retinal ganglion cells. Alternatively, certain injuries to the optic nerve could produce a subtotal but ubiquitous impairment of optic nerve axon conduction. For example, in demyelinating disease high-frequency impulse trains fail to propagate despite the fact that low-frequency impulse trains still conduct reliably (Waxman, 1982). In optic neuropathies there could be an impairment of brightness sense independent of the loss of other visual functions.

These findings corroborate previous studies that demonstrate brightness sense to be an extremely sensitive measure of optic nerve function in patients with optic neuritis and other optic neuropathies (Fleishman et al, 1987; Sadun and Lessell, 1985). Brightness sense was the most sensitive measure among all the visual parameters that we assessed in detecting an optic neuropathy. In some patients with optic neuropathies, particularly those with optic neuritis, brightness sense was the only function that remained impaired. In most other patients it was impaired to a greater extent than visual acuity or color vision.

In this study, color vision as measured with Ishihara or A-O test plates was the least sensitive measure for detecting an optic neuropathy. Although it is true that the Ishihara or A-O test plates are not the most sensitive methods for detecting impairments of color vision (Hart, 1987), they are the most frequently used screening tests for color vision in clinical practice. More extensive and complete measures of color vision might give different results.

Brightness sense values were significantly decreased among all optic neuropathy groups; however, it did not permit differentiation between disease groups. Despite the fact that brightness sense values did not differ significantly by disease status, there emerged certain patterns that assisted in using brightness sense for monitoring optic neuropathies and possibly even in staging optic nerve impairment. A clear-cut correlation exists between severe brightness sense loss and optic disc edema; there is a moderate impairment associated with optic disc atrophy and less severe brightness sense impairment with normal-appearing optic nerve heads. In large part, this may reflect the fact that brightness sense is a functional disorder that is most impaired in the initial stages of an optic neuropathy. A patient with optic neuritis shows the most severe decrement of brightness sense in the acute phase of the disease, which later improves somewhat with resolution of the optic neuritis, even while the optic atrophy persists. Brightness sense does reflect the reversible physiological as well as the irreversible anatomical defect in the optic nerve.

Summary

This study demonstrates that although visual acuity of color vision may be normal, other parameters of vision, most particularly brightness sense, may remain abnormal in patients with optic neuropathies. We suggest that brightness sense be added to the clinician's repertoire of simple tests used in the evaluation of optic nerve function.

Future of the Test

Brightness sense has only recently been undertaken as a means of characterizing and screening for optic neuropathies. We should expect further studies to lead to modifications in the design of the testing method. For example, what would be the effect of testing targets of different sizes? How does brightness sense vary if the target of regard is colored instead of white?

Investigating the kinetics of brightness sense should prove to be another profitable line of study. One great advantage of brightness sense is that since the results are quantitative, the kinetics of brightness sense impairment, or of resolution following changes in light transmission to one eye, can be established. We have noted that patients who have monocular occlusion will temporarily exhibit significant disparity in brightness sense upon removal of this occlusion. This brightness sense disparity is accompanied by an afferent pupillary defect. The afferent pupillary defect resolves in a few minutes; the brightness sense disparity appears to resolve in a few hours. The kinetics of brightness sense can be used to approach issues of dark adaptation or other changes that reflect modulations in retinal sensitivity. Such variations in light sensitivity may be modulated in other parts of the visual system as well.

Finally, brightness sense has been systematically examined in a variety of optic neuropathies and compared with a variety of other visual functions; however, it has not been measured systematically in other ophthalmological diseases. Is brightness sense affected in retinal detachment? What would be the effects of lesions to peripheral retinal versus central retina? Other diseases such as asymmetrical diabetic maculopathies and central serous retinopathy have not yet been assessed for their affect on brightness sense.

In short, since brightness sense is highly sensitive, reliable, and quantitative, it will lend itself well to future investigations into the psychophysics of brightness, the physiology of retinal sensitivity, and the assessment of a wide variety of ophthalmological diseases. We look forward to seeing investigations into these areas.

Summary

Each of these three studies contributes evidence that brightness sense is an important visual function that can be independently quantified. Brightness sense appears to be particularly impaired in patients with optic nerve disease. Like other tests of visual function, brightness sense may be impaired out of proportion to the visual acuity losses in patients with optic neuropathies.

The measurement of brightness sense can be made through a simple device incorporating two sets of polarized lenses. Investigation of brightness sense with this device in normal persons and in patients with optic nerve disease, maculopathies, cataract, and other media opacities show that brightness sense can provide useful information that, in combination with conventional clinical and laboratory investigations, can help lead to an early and accurate diagnosis. Patients with media opacities do not demonstrate any differences in brightness sense. Similarly, patients with factitious visual loss are unable to give reliable differences in brightness sense. Brightness sense impairment is most consistently found in patients with optic neuropathies. Often, brightness sense is the most sensitive technique in establishing the presence of an optic neuropathy and may be the only abnormality noted after resolution of the optic neuropathy.

Although brightness sense is highly sensitive and reliable, it is not specific for particular types of optic neuropathies. Optic disc changes are more useful in characterizing an optic neuropathy. Nonetheless, because of its quantitative nature, brightness sense is very useful in monitoring the course of the patient's illness.

Thus, brightness sense testing is a simple technique providing sensitivity for detecting disease, reliability and specificity for distinguishing between ocular deficits, and quantitative measurement for monitoring the course of ophthalmologic conditions. We suggest that this method will become increasingly important in both clinical and research applications.

References

Berson E. Electrical phenomena in the retina, In Moses RA (ed) Adler's Physiology of the Eye: Clinical Application. St. Louis: CV Mosby Co: 1981;pp. 466-527.

Brown JL, Mueller CG. Brightness discrimination and brightness contrast, In Graham H (ed) Vision and Visual Perception. New York: John Wiley & Sons Inc: 1965;pp. 208-50.

Cornsweet TN. Visual Perception. New York: Academic Press: 1970.

Enoch JM. Quantitative layer-by-layer perimetry. Invest Ophthalmol Vis Sci 1978;17:208-61.

Fleishman JA, Beck RW, Linares OA, Klein JW. Deficits in visual function after resolution of optic neuritis. Ophthalmology 1987;94:1029-35.

Glaser JS. Clinical Evaluation of Optic Nerve Function. Trans Ophthalmol Soc UK 1986;96:359-62.

Hart WM Jr. Acquired dyschromatopsias. Surv Ophthalmol 1987;32:10-31.

Kaufman L. Sight and Mind. An Introduction to Visual Perception. New York: Oxford Univ Press: 1974;pp. 128-52.

Kayama Y, Riso RR, Bartlett JR and Doty RW. Luxotonic Responses of Units in Macaque Striate Cortex. J Neurophysiol 1979;42:1495-1517.

Land EH, McCann JJ. Lightness and retinex theory. J Opt Soc Am 1971;61:1-11.

Mainster M, Diekert JP. A Single Haploscopic Method for quantitating color brightness comparison. Am J Ophthalmol 1980;89(1):58-61.

Preston DS, Bernstein L, Sadun AA. Office Techniques for Detecting Optic Neuropathies: Brightness-Sense compared to Traditional Screening Tests. Neuro-Ophthalmology 1988;8:245-250.

Quigley HA, Addicks EM, Green WR. Optic nerve damage in human glaucoma: III. Quantitative correlation of nerve fiber loss and visual field defect in glaucoma, ischemic neuropathy, papilledema, and toxic neuropathy. Arch Ophthalmol 1982;100:135-46.

Richards JW. Why rods and cones? Biol Cybern 1979;33:125-35.

Rodieck RW. Visual pathways, In Cowan WM, Hall Z, Kandel E (eds) Annual Review of Neuroscience. Palo Alto, Calif: Annual Reviews Inc: 1979;2:193-225.

Rowe MH, Stone J. Naming of neurons: Classification and naming of cat retinal ganglion cells. Brain Behav Evol 1977;14: 185-216.

Sadun AA. The neuroanatomy of the human visual system: Part I - Retinal projections to the LGN and PT as demonstrated with a new stain. Neuro-ophthalmology 1986a;6:353-61.

Sadun AA. Parallel processing in the human visual system: A new perspective. Neuroophthalmology 1986b;6:351-2.

Sadun AA, Johnson BM, Schaecter JD. The neuroanatomy of the human visual system: Part III - Retinal projections to the hypothalamus. Neuro-ophthalmology 1986a;6:371-9.

Sadun AA, Johnson BM, Smith LEH. Neuroanatomy of the human visual system. Part II - Retinal projections to the superior colliculus and pulvinar. Neuro-ophthalmology 1986b;6:363-70.

Sadun AA, Lessell S. Brightness Sense And Optic Nerve Disease. Arch Ophthalmol 103:1985;39-43.

Sadun AA, Schaechter JD. Retinal ganglion axon diameters and their differential distribution to the visual nuclei in man. Invest Ophthalmol Vis Sci 1983;24(suppl):26.

Schiffman HR. Sensation and Perception: An integrated Approach. New York: John Wiley & Sons: 1982.

Sokal RR, Rohlf FJ. Biometry: The Principles and Practice of Statistics in Biological Research, (ed 2,) New York: WH Freeman and Company, 1981.

Von Helmholtz H. Physiological Optics, ed 3, vol 2. Southhall JPC (translated). New York: Dover Publications Inc: 1962.

Wallach H. Brightness constancy and the nature of achromatic colors. J Exp Psychol 1948;38:310-24.

Walsh FB, Hoyt WF. Clinical Neuro-Ophthalmology. Baltimore: Williams & Wilkins Co: 1969; pp. 501-2.

Waxman SG. Membranes, myelin and the pathophysiology of multiple sclerosis. N Engl J Med 1982;306:1529-33.

Weinstein G, Hobson R, Baker F. Extracellular recordings from human retinal ganglion cells. Science 1971;171:1021-4.

Woodworth RS, Schlosberg H. Experimental Psychology. New York: Henry Holt: 1954.

Chapter 3
Critical Flicker Frequency: A New Look at an Old Test

Randall S. Brenton

H. Stanley Thompson

Charles Maxner

Introduction

If a light is repeatedly turned on and off it is seen to flicker, and if it flickers at increasing frequencies, it finally will appear to fuse into a continuous light. At higher frequencies, a subject will perceive the light to be fused as a steady light even though it is still flickering. The threshold at which this illusion can be seen is called critical flicker frequency. This threshold may also be found by decreasing the frequency until the light appears to flicker. The average of the ascending and descending values can be used to approximate the threshold of flicker perception. In the visual system critical flicker frequency, determined in this way, is a test of temporal resolution that is dependent on a subject's conscious determination of threshold.

Critical flicker frequency has gone by a variety of names such as critical flicker fusion and flicker fusion frequency. In this chapter we will use "critical flicker frequency" to refer to related studies in the literature and "foveal flicker fusion frequency" to refer to the testing done in this study using our apparatus. Critical flicker frequency should not be confused with other electrodiagnostic tests such as flicker fusion electroretinogram, photic driving, and flicker visual evoked potentials, and double flash perception.

The pattern reversal visual evoked potential enjoys a certain popularity as an objective indicator of optic nerve dysfunction (Glaser and Laflamme, 1979; Chiappa, 1983; Neima and Regan, 1984; Asselman et al, 1975; Cox et al, 1982). Visual evoked potential testing can detect optic nerve dysfunction in 82% to 100% of patients with optic neuritis (Mathews et al, 1982; Milner et al, 1974). If the visual evoked potential is such a good indicator, why do we need any more tests of optic nerve function? Visual evoked potential testing is expensive, it requires a trained technician, it is time consuming, and it is often disruptive to patient flow in a busy clinic. There are other tests for impaired temporal resolution in optic neuropathy that require less equipment and less technical expertise. One of these is critical flicker frequency. In this chapter we will explain why we chose to go back to critical flicker frequency and then compare critical flicker frequency with visual evoked potential and other tests of optic nerve function.

Historical Background and Literature Review

Critical flicker frequency has been extensively studied during the past century from various points of view. Many of the details are available in reviews (Landis, 1954; Milner et al, 1974; Simonson and Brozek, 1952). We will briefly review the history of critical flicker fusion in clinical testing.

Early flicker studies were done with rotational devices (Landis, 1954) such as a disc with alternating dark and light areas that produced flicker when rotated. Later, shutters were added in front of these discs or in front of other light sources. In the late 1930s, electronic devices with gas discharge tubes were developed. Light-emitting diodes became commercially available in 1969 (Berg and Dean, 1972), and thus only recent studies have utilized them. (Mason et al, 1982; Betta et al, 1983). Rotational and stroboscopic devices were often used in conjunction with white noise generators to mask the auditory cues, but this is not necessary with light-emitting diodes.

The first clinical study of critical flicker frequency was in 1903 by Braunstein (1903). He found that critical flicker fusion was decreased in optic atrophy, retinal disorders, glaucoma, amblyopia, and night blindness. Several authors suggested that flicker fusion phenomena could be used in testing visual fields (Riddell, 1936; Phillips, 1933; Hylkema, 1942; Miles, 1950; Tyler, 1981; Brussell et al, 1982; Overbury et al, 1984). Most of these studies emphasized that critical flicker frequency was abnormal in early or subtle cases of various neuro-ophthalmologic diseases. Aulhorn and Harms (1972) rejected critical flicker frequency as a practical means of visual field testing, citing two main reasons: 1) no specific localizing defect had been shown in a patient who did not also have a similar defect found on carefully performed differential light sensitivity fields, and 2) critical flicker frequency is itself very dependent on light intensity and retinal location. Therefore, it would be difficult to show a defect in flicker sensitivity beyond that accounted for by a defect in light sensitivity. But Patterson et al (1981) showed that temporal resolution loss can be present even when controlling for the loss of differential light sensitivity at the fovea in patients with multiple sclerosis, and there has been a recent renewal of interest in measuring flicker as a visual field test (Tyler, 1981; Brussell et al, 1982; Overbury et al, 1984). However, field testing requires expensive equipment, skilled technicians, and a considerable amount of testing time, so we chose to measure critical flicker fusion at the fovea under photopic conditions (photopic foveal flicker fusion frequency). Most of the optic nerve diseases we wish to detect are characterized by early loss of central visual function and central scotomas, namely, demyelinative and compressive optic neuropathies. Tyler (1981) has used a different flicker phenomenon to measure optic nerve function in glaucoma as a visual field test. This test is called flicker modulation sensitivity. Instead of varying the frequency of on/off cycles, the relative luminance of the on and off periods are changed.

DeLange (1958) produced curves of the attenuation characteristics of white light now called DeLange curves. These curves show that the human visual system is most sensitive to minimal modulation of the stimulus intensity at a level of about 10 Hz. Subsequent authors found the peak sensitivity to be between 10 and 20 Hz (Kelly, 1964). Van der Tweel and Estevez (1974) produced DeLange curves on a patient with optic neuritis and used them to follow the patient's recovery. In the acute phase of optic neuritis, this patient had a severe loss of flicker sensitivity to most frequencies, but after 4 weeks of recovery, flicker modulation sensitivity was depressed primarily at 20 to 30 Hz. Tyler states that flicker modulation sensitivity tested at various frequency levels was more sensitive than critical flicker fusion for detecting glaucomatous damage. Tyler found that when tested centrally, patients with glaucoma produced defects at or below

25 Hz, in the periphery, the defects in flicker modulation sensitivity occurred at greater than 45 Hz or near the maximum found in normal observers. Since he used a relatively large stimulus (5 degrees), they had a relatively high critical flicker frequency in normal subjects (50 Hz). It would be interesting to know if measuring with different stimulus sizes or intensities and producing critical flicker fusion with normal maximal responses at 10 Hz, 20 Hz, 30 Hz, etc. would give a similar response. If the critical flicker frequency normal value was between 20 and 30 Hz, would critical flicker fusion be as sensitive as measuring flicker modulation sensitivity at the same frequencies in optic nerve disease?

Critical flicker frequency has been shown to be abnormal in a high percentage of patients with multiple sclerosis and optic neuritis. Kurachi and Yonemura (1956) found critical flicker frequency to be abnormal in four patients with optic neuritis when using a stimulus of less than 2 degrees of visual angle. Titcombe and Willison (1961) found critical flicker frequency abnormal in 92% (27/29) of patients with multiple sclerosis and a history of optic neuritis and in 51% (16/31) of multiple sclerosis patients without a history of optic neuritis. Parsons and Miller (1957) noted critical flicker frequency to be abnormal in 80% (16/20) of patients with multiple sclerosis. Thorner and Berk (1964) found critical flicker frequency to be abnormal in 96% (58/60) of patients with multiple sclerosis with history of optic neuritis.

Otori et al (1978) found critical flicker frequency to be useful in their neuro-ophthalmology clinic. Unfortunately, their data were not published and no comparisons were made with other standard tests. Namerow (1971), using critical flicker frequency, showed that multiple sclerosis patients were extremely sensitive to raised body temperature.

Critical flicker frequency has failed to become an accepted clinical test despite the glowing reports in the literature. Perhaps there are several reasons for this. No two investigators have used precisely the same technique in clinical trials and thus it is difficult to compare one study with another. Also, there are numerous subject, stimulus, and psychophysical methodologic parameters (Milner et al, 1974; Simonson and Brozek, 1952) that need to be controlled in a given apparatus (see the next section).

One important subject variable is the use of medications: central nervous system stimulants tend to increase the critical flicker frequency and depressants decrease it. Critical flicker frequency is so dependably influenced by drugs that flicker has been used to measure the duration of action of a single dose of diazepam, chlorpromazine, and barbituates (Besser and Duncan, 1967).

Probably the most important reason for the neglect of critical flicker frequency is the advent of various new electrophysiologic tests and psychophysical tests. When it comes to recognizing those patients with optic neuritis who have a prolonged latency of the visual evoked potential, some psychophysical tests, for example, contrast sensitivity with Arden plates (Arden and Gucukaglu, 1978) or double flash perception (Galvin et al, 1976) are no improvement over critical flicker fusion at the fovea. We did a pilot study on patients with recovered optic neuritis and found that critical flicker frequency performed better than Arden contrast sensitivity plates and double flash perception (Brenton et al, 1984). Critical flicker frequency and visual evoked potential were abnormal in 10 of 13 patients with optic neuritis, whereas Arden contrast sensitivity was abnormal in 8 of 13 and double flash perception in 6 of 13.

Parameters and Rationale for Testing Critical Flicker Fusion

The parameters that affect the values of critical flicker frequency include intensity, color, stimulus size, retinal location, retinal adaptation, light-to-dark ratio, method of determining threshold, waveform, pupil and other physiological variables.

Intensity

The intensity of the stimulus is probably the most important testing parameter affecting critical flicker frequency. With increasing intensity, the threshold of critical flicker frequency increases. This relationship is described by the Ferry-Porter law:

$$N = a \log I + b$$

where N = critical flicker frequency in cycles per second, **a** and **b** are constants, and I = intensity of the stimulus.

Since **a** and **b** are constants, this describes a linear relationship, which is true over most of the range of illumination of the fovea (Hecht et al, 1935). Therefore, if the stimulus bulb were to darken with time, critical flicker frequency would change. However, a light-emitting diode's output remains fairly constant for several years. The Ferry-Porter law explains why a patient bothered by the flicker of lights or of a video monitor can be helped by sunglasses. Further, if one is testing with a continuous train of impulses, the mean luminance should be constant so that only the frequency is changed and not both the frequency and the luminance.

Color

Hecht and Shlaer (1936) showed that when stimuli of two different colors are matched for apparent brightness, the critical flicker frequency obtained from each is the same provided the stimulus is in the photopic range. This suggests that the color of the light-emitting diode is not of great importance. We chose to use a red stimulus because it is easily seen and because red has been the most popular stimulus color in previous flicker studies. Furthermore, red light is not blocked as much as shorter wavelengths are by the normal yellowing of the aging lens. Hamano and colleagues (1988) found critical flicker frequency useful for detecting color defects when using stimuli of different colors. For example, protanopia subjects showed a slight decrease in critical flicker frequency using a red stimulus compared with the normal control group, but normal critical flicker frequency using green or yellow. Their subjects with optic neuritis and central serous retinopathy showed profound decreases with all colors. The acquired disorders were easy to separate from the much smaller defects seen with abnormal color vision (Hamano et al, 1988).

Stimulus Size

Stimulus size affects critical flicker frequency especially, with large sized stimuli in the periphery. The Granit-Harper law describes the relationship of flicker frequency to stimulus size (Levinson, 1968):

$$N = a \times \log \text{stimulus area} + b$$

where N = critical flicker frequency in cycles per second, and **a** and **b** are both constants

Critical flicker frequency not only increases with increasing stimulus area, but also varies with retinal locus (Herbolzheimer, 1977). Stimuli of large size tend to have higher critical flicker frequency values in the periphery and small stimuli have higher critical flicker frequency values at the fovea. Theoretically, therefore, an advantage of a small-sized stimulus would be that eccentric fixation would not spuriously lead to elevated readings (Simonson and Brozek, 1952; Hecht and Pirenne, 1933).

Retinal Location

Many studies have been done to determine the effect of different parts of the retina on critical flicker frequency in normal (Herbolzheimer, 1977) and abnormal eyes (Patterson et al, 1981; Braunstein, 1903; Riddell, 1936; Phillips, 1933; Hylkema, 1942; Miles, 1950; Tyler, 1981). With large stimuli, critical flicker frequency increases between 10 and 30 degrees and then decreases toward the periphery (Hartman, 1979). The increase away from the fovea is most pronounced with a stimulus size larger than 5 degrees, which explains why a television set will flicker more when viewed by peripheral retina. We tested eight normal subjects with our apparatus, and eccentric fixation only produced lower critical flicker frequency. This is due to the small stimulus size which tests only cones and to the photopic conditions used for our studies.

Retinal Adaptation

The surrounding illumination influences the level of retinal light adaptation and this influences the critical flicker frequency. With dark adaptation, critical flicker frequency decreases (Lythgoe and Tansley, 1929). Critical flicker frequency is highest when the stimulus is slightly brighter than the surrounding level of illumination (Harvey, 1970). A bright background will also reduce the intersubject variability in pupil size (see "Pupil").

Light-to-Dark Ratio

The ratio of the duration of each brief stimulus to the length of the subsequent dark interval is called the duty cycle. With our instrument, the light interval is kept the same as the dark interval so that the duty cycle is 1.0. Thus the stimulus light is on 50% of the time at all flickering frequencies and a constant mean stimulus intensity is maintained. This helps to avoid changes in the critical flicker frequency due to alteration of the stimulus intensity. Increasing the dark interval relative to the light interval makes the flicker easier to see. Therefore, detection of flicker is more dependent on the dark interval than on the light interval. The Talbot-Plateau law states that the brightness of the light appears to be equivalent to the mean brightness averaged over 1 cycle (Shickman, 1970).

As mentioned previously, the mean luminance should be kept as a constant, if possible, so that only one variable is changed while testing. Maintaining a constant mean stimulus luminance is a problem when measuring flicker modulation sensitivity -- both the luminance of the "on" period and the luminance of the "off" period would need to be changed simultaneously to maintain a constant mean illumination.

Threshold Method

The way in which the threshold frequency is determined can influence the critical flicker fusion measurement. The starting point, rate of change, continuous vs. stair-case technique, and continuous vs. intermittent exposure all influence the results (Simonson and Brozek, 1952; Landis, 1954; Schickman, 1970). A continuous method is used for our testing because it greatly decreases the time required to determine the threshold. Since the eye adapts to flicker, ascending and descending thresholds need to be alternated, or rest periods interspersed, and a relatively constant exposure to the light should be used for all subjects.

Waveform

The waveform is not of great importance in clinical testing because commonly used waveforms (square wave and sinusoidal) have nearly the same physiologic effect (Schickman, 1970; Levinson, 1968). Our apparatus uses a square-wave stimulus.

Pupil

Pupil size is important because it affects the amount of light received by the retina. In general, larger pupils result in a higher critical flicker frequency measure (Simonson and Brozek, 1952; Landis, 1954; Shickman, 1970). In 11 normal subjects we showed that the mean critical flicker fusion frequency was the same for the natural pupil and artificial pupil sizes of 4, 6, and 8 mm. However, critical flicker fusion frequency was 3 Hz lower with a 2mm artificial pupil than with a 4mm pupil (Fig. 3.1). This reduction with a small pupil is probably due to a reduction of retinal illumination. A bright background was used to reduce the variation in pupil sizes between subjects. But if a patient has a small (<2.5 mm) pupil, it may affect the critical flicker frequency. In perimetry, if a small pupil causes a defect, it should be repeated after dilation, and this is a good rule for critical flicker frequency as well.

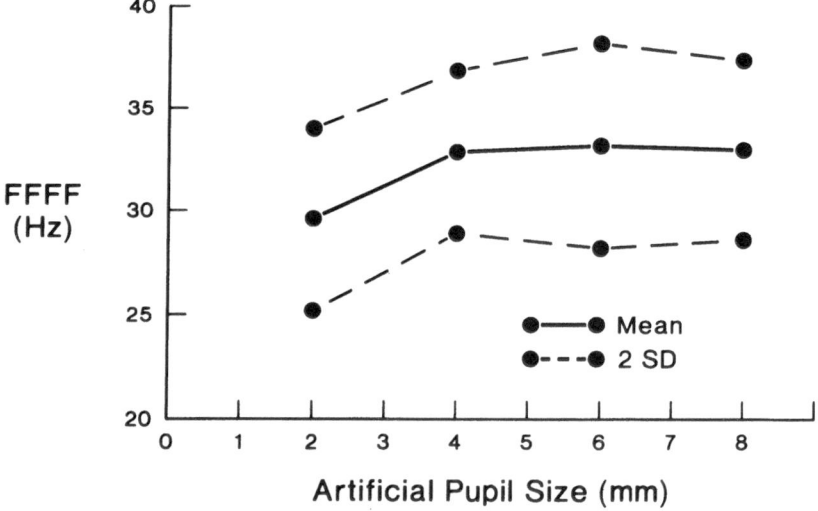

Figure 3.1. Pupil size and foveal flicker fusion frequency in 11 normal subjects tested after dilation with 1% Mydriacyl (tropicamide) and using artificial pupils.

Other Physiologic Variables

A variety of physiologic variables have been found to influence critical flicker frequency: fatigue, age, hypoxia, hypercarbia, acidosis, alkalosis, carbon monoxide poisoning, and numerous medications with central nervous system effects. For further information on the psychophysical and physiologic aspects of critical flicker frequency there are several extensive reviews available (Simonson and Brozek, 1952; Landis, 1954; Shickman, 1970)

Current Studies

Methods Used in Our Clinical Studies

The apparatus constructed at the University of Iowa (Fig. 3.2) uses a red light-emitting diode (Hewlett Packard HLMP-0820) with a peak wavelength of 660 mm, operating at 1.88 mA mounted on a translucent milkglass plate. An incandescent bulb (40 W) is mounted behind this plate with a reflector to give an even illumination of 3.5 candela/m^2 independent of ambient light. The psychophysical impression is that this light-emitting diode is brighter than the surroundings.

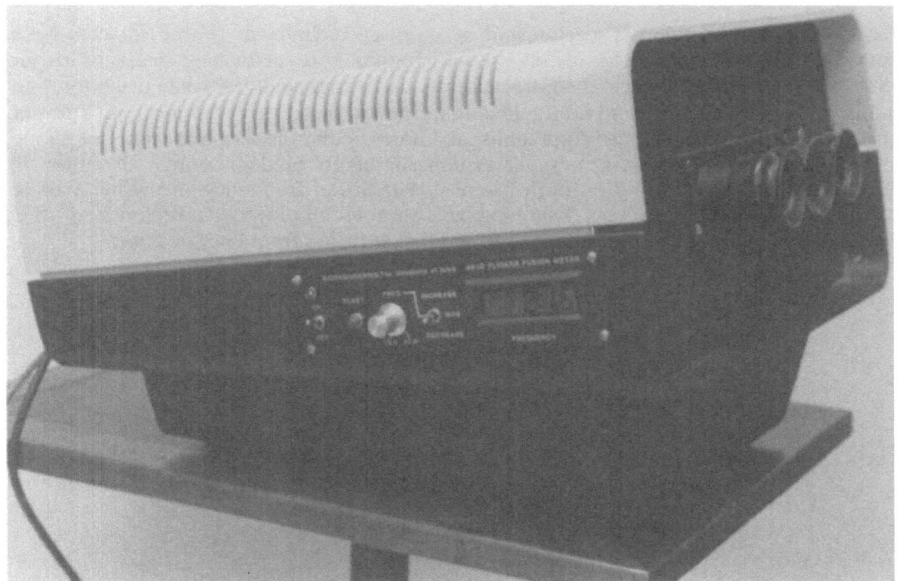

Figure 3.2. The instrument used to determine foveal flicker fusion frequency is shown from the technician's view. The oculars are to the right. The button used by the subject to signal threshold is not shown.

The light-emitting diode subtends 1.4 degrees of arc. An 8 diopter lens is mounted on the ocular 12.5 cm from the diode. The lens places the image at optical infinity and therefore a subject's distance correction can be used. Additional oculars are placed on either side of the central ocular so that during the examination both eyes are exposed to the same background luminance. Baffles mounted in the instrument allow the light-emitting diode to be seen only through the central ocular. The light-emitting diode is connected to a square-wave generator that produces light and dark intervals of equal duration and, therefore, a constant mean illumination at various frequencies. The apparatus produces no audible sounds. The frequency appears on a digital liquid crystal display out of view of the subject. The frequency is changed at a constant rate of 1 Hz automatically by the apparatus with ascending or descending frequencies.

The subject is instructed to fixate on the light-emitting diode while the test is explained and obviously flickering and nonflickering lights are demonstrated. The subject is shown a flickering light and the frequency is then increased at a constant rate (1 Hz) by the machine until the light appears to fuse. At this point, the subject presses a handheld button to record automatically the ascending threshold. The frequency is then increased manually to a point at which it is clearly seen to be fused and is then decreased at a constant rate until the light begins to visibly flicker. The subject then presses the button to automatically record the descending threshold. The mean of these first two measurements, although discarded, serves as a rough estimate of threshold; repeat testing is then performed starting at 10 Hz on either side of this estimate.

Three ascending and three descending measurements are made, and the average of these six values are taken as the foveal flicker fusion frequency for that eye. Testing both eyes takes about 3 minutes.

Control Series

Exactly 103 normal subjects were tested by a novice technician. These subjects were untrained department employees, along with friends and relatives of patients in our clinic waiting room. All normal control subjects had visual acuity of 20/25 or better, had pupils larger than 2.5 mm and no significant anisocoria (more than 0.5 mm), no afferent pupil defect, no current ocular complaints, no known ocular disease, and were not taking medications that were central nervous system stimulants or depressants. Another 50 normal subjects were tested on both foveal flicker fusion frequency and visual evoked potential by trained observers. These subjects were all employees and many had prior testing with visual evoked potential and foveal flicker fusion frequency or both.

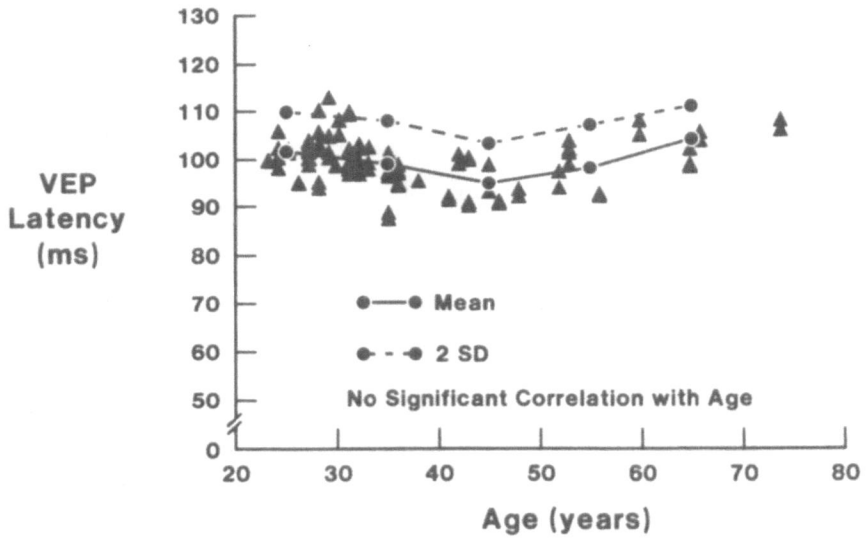

Figure 3.3. Visual evoked potential latency and age were not significantly related in 50 normal volunteers. The mean for the various age groups and the upper limit of normal (2 SD) are shown.

Clinical Studies of Foveal Flicker Fusion Frequency

We compared foveal flicker fusion frequency with several tests that have been used for optic nerve function. Two of these were previously mentioned: Arden contrast sensitivity and double flash perception. After finding foveal flicker fusion frequency superior to these tests, Brenton and colleagues (1984) studied foveal flicker fusion frequency and visual evoked potential, relative afferent pupillary defects (RAPD), American Optical pseudoisochromatic color plates, and foveal differential light threshold as determined on the Humphrey perimeter.

Visual Evoked Potential

Visual evoked potential latency was chosen as a reference test or "gold standard" for comparisons with foveal flicker fusion frequency. The visual evoked potential was obtained using an alternating checkerboard pattern on a television screen subtending 9.5 degrees of visual angle horizontally and 7.5 degrees vertically. The check size was 45 minutes of visual angle with luminance characteristics as described previously (Cox et al, 1982). Pattern reversal rate was 1 Hertz, with 256 reversals being averaged. The visual evoked potential was recorded during monocular stimulation using an electrode montage as previously described (Neima and Regan, 1984).

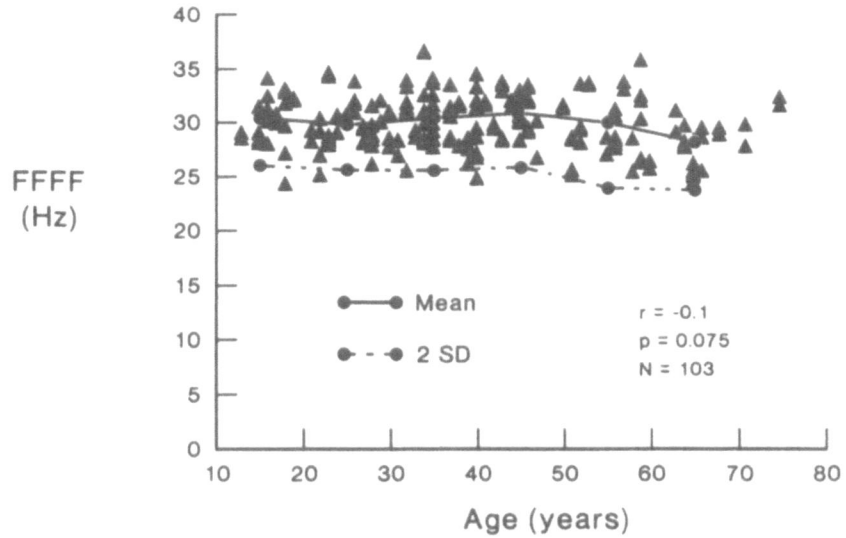

Figure 3.4. Foveal flicker fusion frequency among 103 normal subjects with no prior experience with the test is not significantly related to age. The mean and lower limit of normal (2 SD) are shown for each age group.

Relative Afferent Pupillary Defect

Pupillometer input asymmetry between the two eyes was detected and quantified in each patient using neutral density filters to measure the relative afferent pupillary defect (Thompson and Corbett, 1989).

American Optical Color Plates

Subjects were tested as described in the color plate book. Missing more than four plates was considered abnormal.

Foveal Thresholds

Fifty-three volunteer subjects from the University's eye clinic had the foveal thresholds of both eyes recorded by the Humphrey Field Analyzer. The purpose of the study was to establish the limits of normality for foveal threshold interocular differences. In another study 103 normal subjects had foveal thresholds recorded on the Humphrey Field Analyzer to establish the normal value for a single eye (Brenton and Phelps, 1986).

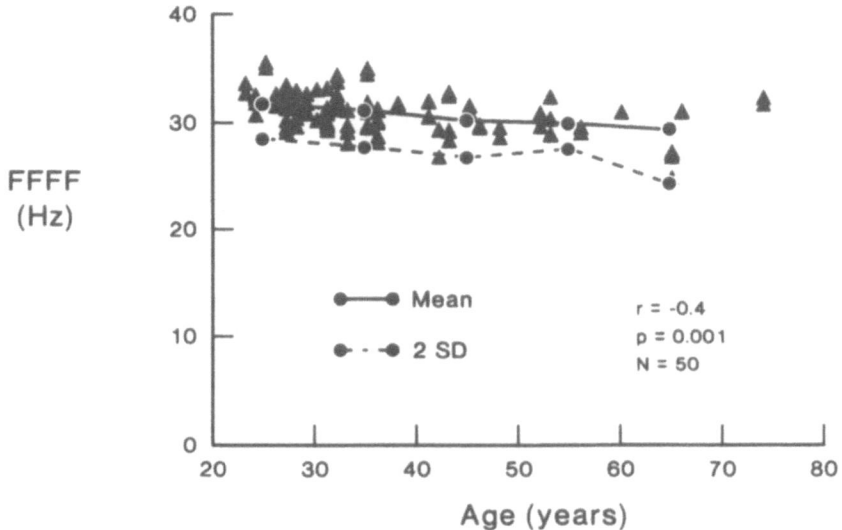

Figure 3.5. Foveal flicker fusion frequency among 50 experienced normal subjects had higher scores than those in Figure 3.3. These were the same subjects tested with visual evoked potential in Figure 3.2. This group of more experienced subjects tested by a trained observer did show a small but significant relationship with age.

Data from Controls

Visual evoked potentials: 50 normal volunteers between the ages of 23 and 75 were tested (mean age = 39.5 years) by a novice observer (Fig. 3.3).

Foveal flicker fusion frequency was not significantly related to age (r = -0.1; P = .075) in this group of first-time subjects (Fig. 3.4). Since previous investigators found a decrease in foveal flicker fusion frequency with age (Glaser and Laflamme, 1979; Chiappa, 1983), we made corrections for age when analyzing patient data. The mean and lower limits of normal (2 SD) are also shown in Figure 3.4 and Table 3.1. The mean interocular difference was 0.5 Hz ±1.8 (SD). These results show wider limits of normality than those obtained by one of us (R.S.B.) on 50 subjects (many having been tested previously) who also had visual evoked potentials performed (Fig. 3.5). The experienced control subject group showed a significant relationship with age as shown in Figure 3.5 (r = 0.4; P <.001). For this group, the intraocular differences were 0.9 Hz ± 0.7. For the analysis of patient data, the novice group of 103 subjects were used for this study, even though the range of normality is greater. We felt that the novice subjects as a control group would better represent the performances of unselected patients. Using an inexperienced technician would also parallel a typical clinical setting.

Foveal Thresholds

Foveal threshold sensitivity was measured in 53 normal subjects with the Humphrey Field Analyzer. Figure 3.6 shows these values, and the limits of normality for this group are in Table 3.1. The range of interocular differences in foveal threshold is shown in Figure 3.7. An interocular difference of 4 dB was considered abnormal. Since these 53 subjects were relatively experienced observers, they were not included with the 103 novice subjects for data analysis.

Table 3.1. Mean and lower limit of normal on 206 eyes for foveal flicker fusion frequency and for 103 eyes for foveal differential light threshold on the Humphrey Field Analyzer

Decade of Age	10-19	20-29	30-39	40-49	50-59	60-69	70+
FFFF(Hz) mean	30.4	29.8	30.4	30.9	30.0	28.2	---
Lower limit of normal (-2 SD)	26.0	25.6	25.6	25.9	24.4	23.8	---
N =	24	34	52	40	32	24	---
Foveal mean	---	37.6	37.2	35.7	36.3	35.2	34.5
Threshold lower limit of normal (dB) (-2 SD)	---	34.6	33.0	32.5	33.1	31.0	29.9
N =	---	17	18	18	18	18	13

Data on the foveal threshold are from a separate study (Brenton and Phelps, 1986).

Patient Studies

The first clinical study consisted of 51 patients with various optic nerve diseases tested with both visual evoked potential and foveal flicker fusion frequency. All of these subjects had a clearly established clinical diagnosis. Twenty-seven patients had optic neuritis, 10 patients had other optic neuropathies, and 14 patients had pseudotumor cerebri without optic neuropathy. None of the patients were taking medications that would alter their test performance.

The second clinical study was a study of consecutive patients seen in the neuro-ophthalmology clinic. In this study 186 eyes were tested. All the subjects had 20/400 Snellen acuity or better but were otherwise unselected and represented a sample of con-

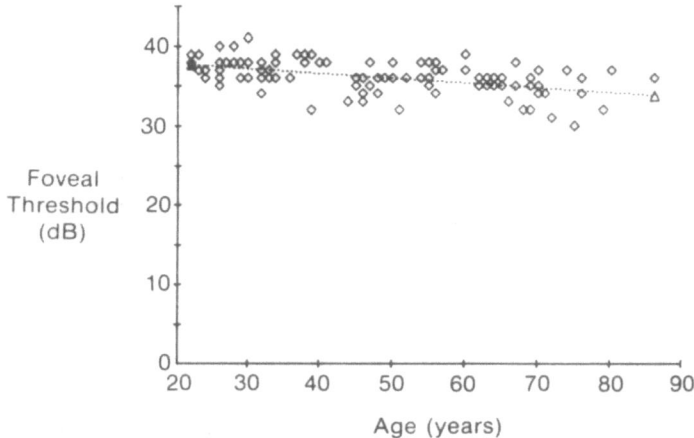

Figure 3.6. Fifty-three normal subjects tested for foveal threshold on the Humphrey Field Analyzer.

secutive patients seen in our neuro-ophthalmology clinic. American Optical pseudoisochromatic color plate scores were determined and considered abnormal if there were five errors for a given eye or a difference of more than two plates between eyes.

A final clinical study was a comparison of foveal flicker fusion frequency and foveal thresholds on the Humphrey Field Analyzer obtained in 53 eyes of patients seen in the neuro-ophthalmology clinic. This group includes some of the subjects from the second clinical study group (sensitivity/specificity). There is a selection bias in this final group because subjects being tested for foveal thresholds usually were suspected of having optic neuropathy.

Foveal Flicker Fusion Frequency vs. Visual Evoked Potential in Optic Neuritis

Twenty-seven patients with optic neuritis were studied; six patients had bilateral disease for a total of 33 affected eyes. Of the affected eyes 63% had 20/20 or better acuity, with the worst visual acuity being 20/70. Most of the affected eyes were in various stages of recovery, from days to several years after onset Of the 33 eyes tested, 82% (27/33) had abnormal foveal flicker fusion frequency values and 88% (29/33) had abnormal visual evoked potential latencies by using 1) the score for the affected eye or 2) the interocular difference. Three eyes were normal by both tests.

Of the 33 affected eyes, three were excluded from further analysis because of either nonrecordable visual evoked potential (two cases) or nonrecordable foveal flicker fusion frequency (one case). Figure 3.8 shows the relation between the foveal flicker fusion frequency and visual evoked potential latency in the 30 remaining eyes with optic neuritis. There is a high degree of correlation (r = -0.7, P <.001).

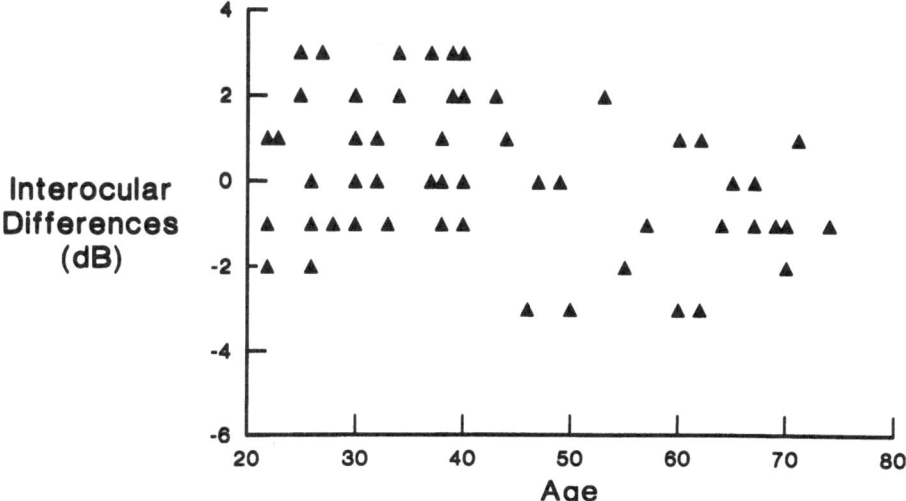

Figure 3.7. The interocular differences (right eye-left eye) of the 53 normal subjects shown in Figure 3.5. We concluded from this that an interocular difference of 4 dB or more might be considered abnormal.

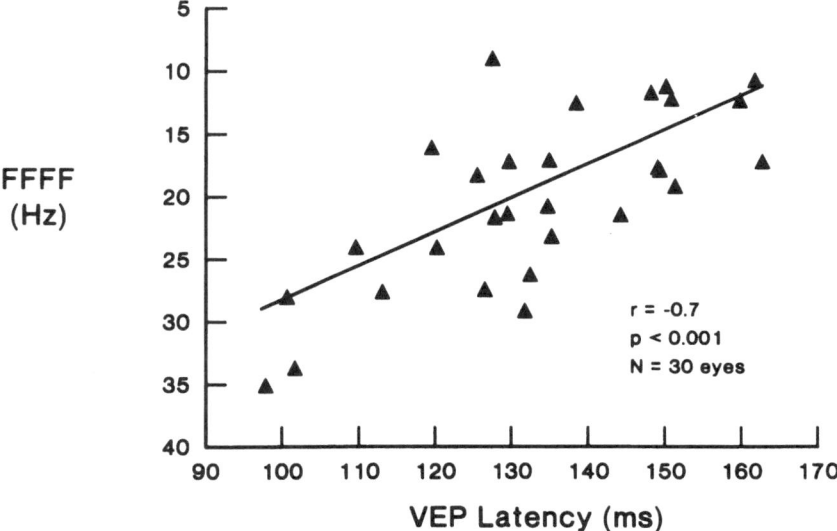

Figure 3.8. Visual evoked potential latency and foveal flicker fusion frequency in 30 eyes with optic neuropathy in various stages of recovery.

In 22 patients with either a completely unilateral optic neuritis or a clearly asymmetric involvement in bilateral cases, we compared the difference between the two eyes. Figure 3.9 shows the interocular differences of foveal flicker fusion frequency and visual evoked potential latency. This relationship, although not as close, is also significant (r = 0.48, P <.05).

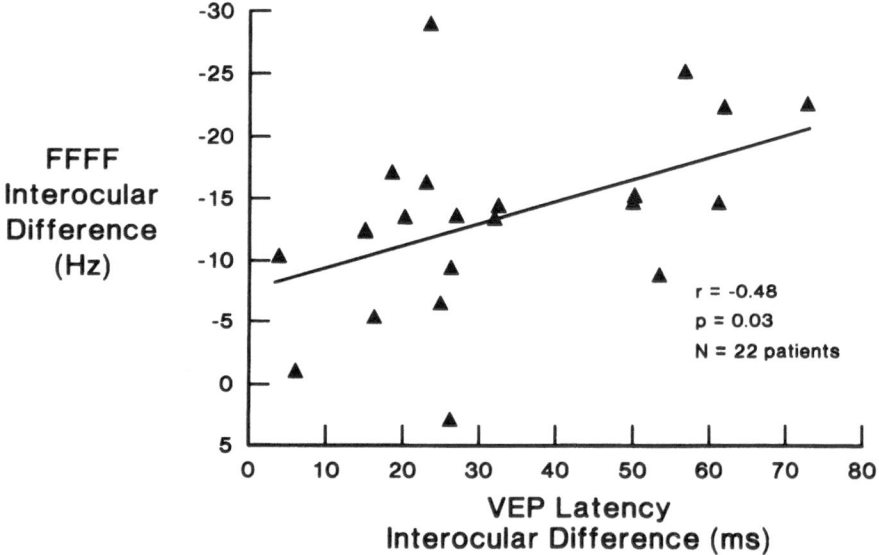

Figure 3.9. The difference between the two eyes of foveal flicker fusion frequency and visual evoked potential latency shows a good correlation among these 22 patients with apparently asymmetric optic neuritis.

Foveal Flicker Fusion Frequency vs. Relative Afferent Pupillary Defect in Optic Neuritis

There were 18 patients with strictly unilateral involvement. Figure 3.10 shows the plot of the regression line for the patient's foveal flicker fusion frequency value (interocular difference) versus the patient's relative afferent pupillary defect measured in log units. When a neutral density filter is held in front of a normal eye just before the foveal flicker fusion frequency is measured, the fusion frequency drops about 2 Hz for every 0.3 log of filter (dashed line in Fig. 3.10).

Of these 18 patients, three had no relative afferent pupillary defect and two had normal foveal flicker fusion frequency. Because relative afferent pupillary defect is a comparison between the two eyes, it is valuable when dealing with purely unilateral disease. As we will see in later studies, however, the relative afferent pupillary defect may be absent in bilateral symmetric disease, and it may fail to detect the less involved eye in patients with slightly asymmetric visual evoked potentials.

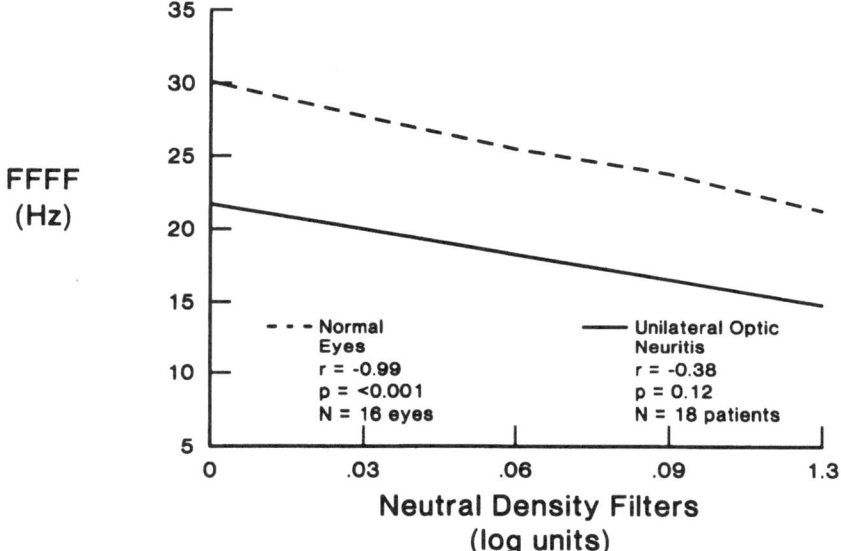

Figure 3.10. The correlation of foveal flicker fusion frequency with afferent pupil defects in log units did not reach statistical significance (solid line). However, this relationship paralleled the relationship of foveal flicker fusion frequency decrease by light attenuation. The flicker fusion frequency decrease caused by light attenuation in normal eyes is shown by the dashed line.

Foveal Flicker Fusion Frequency vs. Visual Evoked Potential in Other Optic Neuropathies

In another group of patients with other optic neuropathies that commonly cause loss of central vision, a similar high correlation between foveal flicker fusion frequency and visual evoked potential latencies ($r = -0.68$; $P < .05$) was found (Fig. 3.11). Figure 3.11 includes two eyes with Graves' optic neuropathy, two eyes with compressive optic neuropathy from frontal mucocele, two eyes with traumatic optic neuropathy, two eyes with dominant optic atrophy, and two eyes with idiopathic optic atrophy.

A diminished foveal flicker fusion frequency is not a specific sign of optic nerve disease. Macular disease also lowers the foveal flicker fusion frequency. It is one of several "optic nerve function tests" known to be abnormal in patients with retinal disease (Hecht and Shlaer, 1936; Folk et al, 1984; Alkhomis and Easterbrook, 1983).

To assess for false positive results, we studied a group of patients with pseudotumor cerebri and no evidence of optic nerve dysfunction (normal visual evoked potential, normal visual field, and no afferent pupil defect). All 14 patients had normal foveal flicker fusion frequency scores in both eyes.

Sensitivity and Specificity of Foveal Flicker Fusion Frequency,
Pseudoisochromatic Plates and Relative Afferent Pupillary Defect.

When evaluating a clinical test, two pieces of information are vital. The first -- called specificity -- is the likelihood that a positive result indicates disease (true positives divided by the sum of true positives and false positives). The second -- called sensitivity -- is the likelihood that a patient with a disease will have a positive test (true positives divided by the sum of true positives and false negatives). Sensitivity and specificity must be considered in a defined population. For many authors, this population is defined by which patients were tested in a selected fashion. Christ et al,(1986) recently proposed a new test of optic nerve function. They asked patients to match the luminance of a steady light to that of a flickering light. They found that 24 of 25 cases had abnormal results and thus the test had 96% sensitivity. These patients all had decreased visual acuity, central scotomas, and prolonged visual evoked potential latencies. To be of clinical value, a test must retain its sensitivity under adverse conditions; for example, it must be able to identify minimal disease. Our test of foveal flicker fusion frequency retained a sensitivity of 82% in recovered optic neuritis (63% of the group had normal visual acuity). To give a true indication of the sensitivity and specificity of a test, one must test a number of consecutive patients in a defined clinical population, so that subjects with a variety of diseases may be tested.

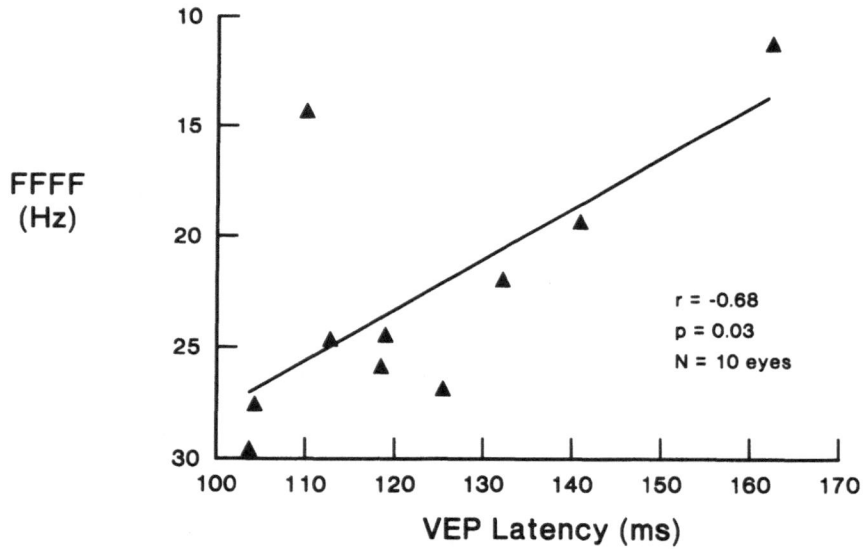

Figure 3.11. Foveal flicker fusion frequency visual evoked potential were significantly related among patients with various optic neuropathies that tend to produce loss of vision centrally.

The 186 eyes of 93 consecutive Neuro-Ophthalmology Clinic patients were used to assess the sensitivity and specificity of this test in this study population. The subjects almost always had American Optical color plate scores recorded and

Table 3.2. Diagnostic groups for sensitivity and specificity studies of foveal flicker fusion frequency

Category	Disease	Number
I (Normal vision)	Normal*	45
	Graves' without neuropathy	18
	PTC without neuropathy	5
	Migraine	9
	Diplopia	11
	Other	23
		111
II (Ocular disease affecting vision)	Amblyopia	4
	Uveitis	5
	Cataracts	3
	Other	6
		18
III (Disc-Related optic nerve head damage)	Ischemic optic neuropathy	4
	Glaucoma	4
	PTC with active neuropathy	1
		9
IV (Optic neuropathy) compressive	Demyelinative	12
	Graves'	12
	Chiasmal	10
	Other	14
		48
TOTAL:		186

* Many of these are fellow eyes in patients with one of the other diseases.
PTC = pseudotumor cerebri

always had a pupil examination for afferent pupillary defects. The data were analyzed on the basis of whether a test result was normal or abnormal. The subjects were divided into four diagnostic groups, as shown in Table 3.2. Patients in category I had either normal eye examination findings or an ocular problem not affecting the vision at the time of the examination. Category II includes patients that had altered vision but no optic nerve disease. Category III patients had optic neuropathy that caused optic nerve head damage or disc-related visual loss. Patients in category IV had optic neuropathies tending to produce loss of central vision.

The results of the sensitivity/specificity study are shown in Table 3.3 and Table 3.4. The data were analyzed in three diagnostic categories. A subgroup of category IV consists of acute cases of optic neuropathy (Table 3.3). Among these subjects foveal flicker fusion frequency performed the best, with 95% sensitivity. When considering all category IV subjects (both acute and chronic optic neuropathies), foveal flicker fusion frequency was still the best of the three tests listed. Certainly the numbers for relative afferent pupillary defects were affected by the fact that this test is only useful in asymmetric disease and would, therefore, miss any cases that were bilaterally symmetric. The better eye was not included in this table for relative rfferent pupillary defects in asymmetric disease, possibly giving a bias toward improved sensitivity of the relative afferent pupillary defect test.   Finally, when considering any optic neuropathy, the afferent pupil defect performed the best.   Unfortunately, visual evoked potential testing was not performed on this entire group of consecutive patients because of the inability of our laboratory to handle this number of patients.

Table 3.3. Sensitivity and specificity data of foveal flicker fusion frequency

	Acute		Category IV		Category III & IV (combined)	
	Optic Neuropathies (subset of category IV)		Optic Neuropathies (acute & recovered)		All Optic Neuropathies (including nerve head disease)	
	Sens	Spec	Sens	Spec	Sens	Spec
RAPD[*]	88%[+]	27%[+]	68%	65%	74%	92%
AO plates	81%	29%	61%	48%	63%	59%
FFFF	95%	43%	77%	80%	68%	85%

[*] Eyes that could have RAPD. Includes only unilateral cases, i.e., cases in which the affected eyes could be compared with a normal eye. In bilateral cases the less involved eye was excluded.
[+] Inaccurate because of small numbers (N = 7)
RAPD = relative afferent pupillary defect, FFFF = foveal flicker fusion frequency

Foveal Flicker Fusion Frequency vs. Foveal Thresholds in Compressive or Demyelinative Optic Neuropathy

The study of 51 patients with foveal flicker fusion frequency and foveal differential light sensitivity is shown in Table 3.5. Eyes listed as normal had no visual disturbance but there may have been something wrong with the other eye. Eyes shown as having an ocular disease include patients with disc-related optic neuropathies (although they didn't necessarily have disc-related visual field loss in every case). The 22 eyes labeled retrobulbar optic neuropathy had either retrobulbar optic neuritis or compressive optic neuropathy. Visual acuity was defined as normal if it was 20/25 or better. One normal subject was abnormal on foveal threshold testing, but this value was only slightly outside the 95% confidence interval. Foveal flicker fusion frequency detected optic neuropathies better than visual acuity testing or foveal threshold testing.

Discussion

Foveal flicker fusion frequency shows a good correlation with visual evoked potential latency in patients with minimal decrease in vision due to optic neuritis and other optic neuropathies and it is clearly abnormal in cases of recovered optic neuritis with normal acuity and no clinically detectable visual field defects. Thus, foveal flicker fusion frequency is useful in confirming the presence of optic nerve dysfunction and is a good predictor of visual evoked potential latency in optic neuropathy. Very few subjects had normal foveal flicker fusion frequency and abnormal visual evoked potential latency and vice versa (Fig. 3.8).

Table 3.4. Abnormal values

Category	I Normal		II Ocular Disease		III Disc-Related Neuropathy		IV Other Optic Neuropathy	
	N	Abn	N	Abn	N	Abn	N	Abn
RAPD*	111	2%	15	20%	7	100%	28	68%
AO plates	99	11%	18	56%	7	86%	44	61%
FFFF	111	2%	18	33%	9	23%	48	77%

* Includes only unilateral disease, i.e., cases in which the affected eye could be compared with a normal eye. In bilateral cases the less involved eye was excluded (not the same patients as RAPD).
Abbreviations are explained in Table 3.3 footnote.

It is well known from visual evoked potential latency work that optic neuritis can cause a striking delay of transmission well beyond that which can be accounted for by simple light attenuation. It is generally accepted that this delay is due to impaired optic nerve conduction resulting from patchy demyelination. A parallel striking loss of temporal resolution in optic neuritis can be demonstrated with foveal flicker fusion frequency (Figs. 3.8, 3.9 and Table 3.5). The further decrease of foveal flicker fusion frequency with increasing afferent pupillary defects in asymmetric optic neuritis (Fig. 3.10) parallels the decrease due to light attenuation.

A review of all factors that might alter foveal flicker fusion frequency (Simonson and Brozek, 1952; Landis, 1954; Shickman, 1970) might lead to the conclusion that foveal flicker fusion frequency is subject to a large number of false positive results. Our testing apparatus controls for most of these factors, and there were no false positives among 14 patients with pseudotumor cerebri without optic neuropathy. Further, patients on medications or with medical conditions that might alter their performance on psychophysical tests would be expected to perform poorly with both eyes. But using criteria of interocular differences in asymmetric optic neuritis, the more severely affected eye (as defined by symptoms and visual acuity) was identified in 20 of 22 (91%) cases. Although the correlation of foveal flicker fusion frequency interocular differences with visual evoked potential latency interocular differences is not as high as that for the score of the affected eye alone, this criterion for abnormality is quite helpful in asymmetric disease.

Table 3.5. Foveal thresholds vs.
foveal flicker fusion frequency

	Normal Eyes (N = 25)	Ocular Disease [*] (N = 6)	Retrobulbar Optic Neuropathy [+] (N = 22)
	Abnormal		
Visual acuity (> than 20/25)	0%	33%	55%
FFFF	0%	33%	91%
Foveal threshold	4%	33%	59%

[*] Includes disc-related optic neuropathy.
[+] Includes compression and demyelination.

In our small group of eyes with other optic neuropathies (compressive optic neuropathy, traumatic optic neuropathy, dominant optic atrophy, idiopathic optic atrophy) the foveal flicker fusion frequency again correlated well with the visual evoked potential latency (Fig. 3.11). These disorders tend to produce central visual loss and therefore would cause significant reductions in the foveal flicker fusion frequency. We only tested foveal function, but others (Riddell, 1936; Phillips, 1933; Hylkema, 1942; Miles, 1950; Tyler, 1981) have found early loss of temporal resolution with flicker phenomenon in the visual periphery in diseases that cause early loss in the periphery, such as glaucoma. Because of problems with increased testing time, equipment costs, and correcting for differences in luminance at different retinal eccentricities, the use of critical flicker fusion in visual field testing is not as handy a clinical tool as foveal testing.

The data from the 186 eyes in the sensitivity/specificity study (Table 3.3) show that foveal flicker fusion frequency is very sensitive for acute optic neuropathies and both sensitive and specific for demyelinative/compressive optic neuropathies. American Optical pseudoisochromatic color plates are less sensitive and less specific for all categories of optic nerve disease. The relative afferent pupil defect is more sensitive for detecting unilateral ocular disease and less specific for optic neuropathies than foveal flicker fusion frequency. There is considerable bias when looking at the afferent pupil defect in this way because it only tells us about asymmetric disease. It is usually easy to recognize a problem with the more affected eye, but relatively more difficult to detect abnormality of the less affected fellow eye in bilateral disease. No similar study of visual evoked potential has been performed to measure its sensitivity and specificity within a defined population base.

Foveal flicker fusion frequency was able to detect optic neuropathy in patients in whom automated static perimetry found no central scotoma. Foveal threshold testing detected a subtle central deficit often not found on confrontation or Goldmann visual fields. Several patients had normal foveal thresholds and clearly abnormal foveal flicker fusion frequency.

Foveal flicker fusion frequency was most useful in detecting acute optic neuropathies due to demyelinative or compressive lesions. But the sensitivity/specificity data do not reflect foveal flicker fusion frequency value in other diseases.

In an unpublished study of 13 patients with Graves' compressive optic neuropathy, we found that foveal flicker fusion frequency performed as well as visual evoked potential (Brenton et al, 1984). Eight patients had bilateral disease. Many of the affected eyes were tested more than once for a total of 37 visits. Foveal flicker fusion frequency was abnormal in 68% of visits (25/37) and visual evoked potential was abnormal in 73% (27/33). At the first visit of the 21 affected eyes, foveal flicker fusion frequency was abnormal in 67% (14/21) and visual evoked potential was abnormal in 67% (14/21). However, foveal flicker fusion frequency and visual evoked potential were not always abnormal for the same eyes. If the two tests are combined, one of the two tests was abnormal in 90% (19/21) of the affected eyes. In the case of Graves' compressive optic neuropathy, foveal flicker fusion frequency seems to give additional information to the visual evoked potential in some patients.

In a study of patients with central serous retinopathy Folk and colleagues (1984) found that afferent pupil defects and foveal flicker fusion frequency are the first tests to return to normal after resolution of central serous retinopathy and visual acuity. Visual evoked potential latency and FM-100 scores improve later. Therefore, foveal flicker fusion frequency may help to distinguish recovering central serous retinopathy from optic neuritis.

Suggestible patients with functional visual loss may give normal foveal flicker fusion frequency responses. But many show an unusually large variability in the ascending and descending thresholds. Several patients who believed their right eye to be blind put their eyes to the left pair of oculars and, believing that the left eye was being tested, gave an entirely normal response.

Cataracts can decrease foveal flicker fusion frequency. Patients with visual acuity of 20/40 or worse because of cataracts will probably have an abnormal foveal flicker fusion frequency. A study of a large number of patients with various types of media opacities has not been done. But as a rule, if there is a clinically obvious media opacity and foveal flicker fusion frequency is decreased, one should blame the media opacity.

Foveal flicker fusion frequency can be affected anywhere along the visual pathway, except it does not seem to be affected by small refractive errors. Foveal flicker fusion frequency is most helpful when eye examination findings are normal and an optic nerve problem is suspected clinically.

If the visual evoked potential latency is more objective, and perhaps more specific for optic nerve deficits, is there a need for another optic nerve test? We think that foveal flicker fusion frequency serves a useful purpose in our clinic for several reasons. The visual evoked potential is a very expensive test requiring a full-time trained technician, whereas foveal flicker fusion frequency can be performed either by the clinician or by an assistant in minutes and the apparatus costs relatively little. The visual evoked potential equipment is not portable and is not readily available to many ophthalmologists. Foveal flicker fusion frequency is very quick and does not slow down the evaluation of patients, as would scheduling electrophysiologic testing. Because of its simplicity, speed, and ease of testing for patients, and because of its good correlation with visual evoked potential latency, it is a useful tool for detecting optic nerve dysfunction even when other measures such as visual acuity are normal. This test has gained favor in our neuro-ophthalmology clinic and has become a routine part of our evaluation of optic nerve function.

Future of the Test

Patients with suppression amblyopia are currently being examined with Foveal flicker fusion frequency in a multicenter study. Patients with amblyopia sometimes show a "better" than normal response. Eccentric fixation alone does not account for this observation, and it is hoped that flicker fusion thresholds may shed some light on the pathophysiology of amblyopia.

Foveal flicker fusion is now being used in several centers as a routine clinical test of optic nerve function. An instrument is not currently being commercially marketed, although similar devices have been made and sold in Japan. Routine use of this test in a clinical setting by clinicians will ultimately determine whether the test earns widespread acceptance.

Summary

Foveal flicker fusion frequency is a psychophysical test of visual temporal resolution. It is a test that is easy to perform, inexpensive, and gives reproducible results. It is a useful clinical tool because it has a high correlation with pattern reversal visual evoked potential latency in patients with recovering optic neuritis (r = -0.8, P <.001) and in patients with other optic neuropathies (r = -0.7, P <.05). Foveal flicker fusion frequency may be abnormal in a number of ophthalmic disorders. It is especially useful in Graves' optic neuropathy. Although foveal flicker fusion frequency can be abnormal in diseases causing disc-related visual loss (pseudotumor cerebri, glaucoma, and anterior ischemic optic neuropathy), it is not as sensitive as other standard clinical tests for these conditions, but this information may be helpful in the differential diagnosis of these diseases.

References

Alkhomis AR, Easterbrook M. Critical flicker fusion frequency in early chloroquine retinopathy. Can J Ophthalmol 1983;18:217-9.

Arden GB, Gucukaglu AG. Grating test of contrast sensitivity in patients with retrobulbar neuritis. Arch Ophthalmol 1978;96:1626-8.

Asselman P, Chadwick DW, Marsden DD. Visual evoked response in the diagnosis and management of patients suspected of multiple sclerosis. Brain 1975;98:261-82.

Aulhorn E, Harms H. Visual perimetry. In: Jameson D, Hurvich LM (eds) Handbook of Sensory, Physiology, Visual Psychophysics, vol VII 14. New York:Springer-Verlag:1972.

Berg A, Dean P. Light-emitting diodes. Institute of Electrical and Electronics Engineers Proceedings, 1972.

Besser GM, Duncan C. The time course of action of single doses of diazepam, chlopromazine, and some barbituates as measured by auditory flicker fusion and visual flicker fusion thresholds in man. Br J Pharmacol Chemother 1967;30:341-8.

Betta A, DeSanta A, Saronitto C, D'Ardrea F. Flicker fusion test and occupational toxicology: Performance evaluation in workers exposed to lead and solvents. Human Toxicol 1983;2:83-90.

Braunstein EP. Beitrug zuer Lehre des intermittieren der lichtreizes der gesunden and kranken retina. Physiol 1903;33:p. 171.

Brenton RS, Phelps CD. The normal field on the Humphrey field analyzer. Ophthalmologica 1986;193:56-74.

Brenton RS, Thompson HS, Musser C. Flicker fusion as an indicator of optic nerve function. Unpublished data (1984) available on request from: C.S. O'Brien Library, Dept. of Ophthalmology, University of Iowa Hospitals, Iowa City, Iowa 52242.

Brussell EM, White CW, Bross M, et al. Multi-flash campimetry in multiple sclerosis. Curr Eye Res 1981/82;1:671-77.

Chiappa HK. Evoked Potentials in Clinical Medicine. New York: Raven Press:1983.

Christ T, Stodtmeister R, Pillunat L. The flicker test according to Aulhorn. A new method in the diagnosis of optic neuritis In Smith JL (ed) Neuro-ophthalmology Now. New York:Field, Rich and Associates, Inc.:1986.

Cox TA, Thompson HS, Hayreh SS, et al. Visual evoked potential and pupillary signs. A comparison in optic nerve disease. Arch Ophthalmol 1982;100:1603-7.

deLange DZN. Research into the dynamic nature of the human fovea cortex systems with intermittent and modulated light. I. attenuation characteristics with white and colored light. J Opt Soc Am 1958;48:777-84.

Folk JC, Thompson HS, Han DP, et al. Visual function abnormalities in central serous retinopathy. Arch Ophthalmol 1984;102:1299-1302.

Galvin RJ, Regan D, Heron JR. Impaired temporal resolution of vision after acute retrobulbar neuritis. Brain 1976;99:255-68.

Glaser JS, Laflamme P. The visual evoked response: Methodology and application in optic nerve disease. In Thompson HS (ed) Topics in Neuro-Ophthalmology. Baltimore: Williams & Wilkins:1979.

Hamano K, Miyamoto T, Nagai M, et al. Critical flicker frequencies. In Venrost G (ed) Doc Ophthalmol Proc Ser 46. Colour Vision Deficiencies VIII. Proceedings of the International Symposium Avignon. Boston:D.W. Junk Publishers:1988

Hartman E, Lachenmayr B, Brettel H. The peripheral critical flicker frequency. Vis Res 1979;19:1019-23.

Harvey LO. Flicker sensitivity and apparent brightness as a function of surround luminance. J Opt Soc Am 1970;40:860-4.

Hecht S, Pirenne MH. Intermittent stimulation by light. III, The relationship between intensity and critical fusion frequency for different retinal locations. J Gen Physiol 1933;17:251.

Hecht S, Shlaer S. Intermittent stimulation by light. I, The relation between intensity and critical frequency for different parts of the spectrum. J Gen Physiol 1936;19:965-79.

Hecht S, Shlaer S, Smith EL. Intermittent light stimuli and the duplicity theory of vision. Cold Spring Harbor Symp Quant Biol 1935;3:237-44.

Herbolzheimer W. The effect of area on the critical flicker threshold. Albrecht Von Graefes Arch Klin Exp Ophthalmol 1977;204:73-8.

Hylkema BS. Examination of the visual field by determining the fusion frequency. Acta Ophthalmol 1942;20:181-93.

Kelly DH. Sine waves and flicker fusion. Proc Symp Physiology of Flicker. Doc Ophthalmol 1964;18:16.

Kurachi Y, Yonemura D. Critical fusion frequency in retrobulbar neuritis. Arch Ophthalmol 1956;55:371-9.

Landis C. Determinants of the critical flicker fusion threshold. Physiol Rev 1954;34:259-86.

Levinson JZ. Flicker fusion phenomenon. Science 1968;160:21-8.

Lythgoe RJ, Tansley K. The adaptation of the eye: its relation to the critical frequency of flicker. Med Res Counc Spec Rep Ser No 134, 1929.

Mason RJ, Snelgon RS, Foster DH, et al. Abnormalities of chromatic and luminance critical flicker frequency in multiple sclerosis. Invest Ophthalmol Vis Sci 1982;23:246-52.

Mathews WB, Small DG, Small M, Pountney E. Pattern reversal evoked visual potential in the diagnosis of multiple sclerosis. J Neurol Neurosurg Psychiatr 1982;40:1009-14.

Miles PW. Flicker fusion fields. II Findings in early glaucoma. Arch Ophthalmol 1950;43:661-77.

Milner BA, Regan D, Heron JR. Differential diagnosis of multiple sclerosis by visual evoked potential recording. Brain 1974;97:755-72.

Namerow NS. Temperature effect on critical flicker fusion in multiple sclerosis. Arch Neurol 1971;25:269-75.

Neima D, Regan D. Pattern visual evoked potentials and spatial vision in retrobulbar neuritis and multiple sclerosis. Arch Neurol 1984;41:198-201.

Otori T, Hohki T, Nakao Y. Central critical fusion frequency in neuro-ophthalmologic practice. Doc Ophthalmol Proc Ser 1978;19:95-9.

Overbury O, Brussell EM White, CW, et al. Evaluating visual loss with multi-flash campimetry. Can J Ophthalmol 1984;19:253-60.

Parsons OA, Miller PN. Flicker fusion thresholds in multiple sclerosis. Arch Neurol Psychiatr 1957;77:134-9.

Patterson VA, Foster DH, Heron JR, et al. Multiple sclerosis: luminance threshold and measurements of temporal characteristics of vision. Arch Neurol 1981;38:687-89.

Phillips G. Perception of flicker in lesions of the visual pathways. Brain 1933;56:464-78.

Riddell LA. The use of the flicker phenomenon in the investigation of the field of vision. Br J Ophthalmol 1936;20:385-410.

Shickman GM. Time-dependent functions in vision. In Moses RA (ed) Adlers Physiology of the Eye, ed 5. St. Louis: C.V. Mosby:1970.

Simonson E, Brozek J. Flicker fusion frequency background and applications. Physiol Rev 1952;32:349-78.

Thompson HS, Corbett JJ. In defense of the alternating light test (letter to the editor) Neurology 1989;39:154-8.

Thorner MW, Berk MF. Flicker fusion test in neuro-ophthalmologic conditions including multiple sclerosis. Arch Ophthalmol 1964;71:897-915.

Titcombe AF, Willison RG. Flicker fusion in multiple sclerosis. J Neurol Neurosurg Psychiat. 1961;24:260-5.

Tyler CW. Specific deficits at flicker sensitivity in glaucoma and ocular hypertension. Invest Ophthalmol Vis Sci 1981;20:204-12.

van der Tweel LH, Estevez O. Subjective and objective evaluation of flicker. Doc Ophthalmol 1974;169:70-1.

Chapter 4
Contrast Sensitivity Testing

Mark J. Kupersmith

Karen Holopigian

William H. Seiple

Introduction

The detection of small luminance differences between objects and their backgrounds is an important tool for navigating in the visual environment. Many visual system disorders cause patients to complain that their vision is cloudy or blurred, or that the borders of objects are blurred, even though they retain 20/20 Snellen acuity. These patients may suffer from losses in contrast sensitivity that cannot be detected using standard clinical testing. A more appropriate measure for these patients is their ability to detect small changes in luminance within a pattern. One widely used experimental measure of this ability is the contrast sensitivity function.

Operationally, a contrast threshold sensitivity refers to the minimum difference in luminance necessary for an observer to reliably detect an edge. A contrast sensitivity function is a plot of the minimum contrast necessary for detection of objects and patterns over a range of various retinal image sizes. Since Campbell and Green (1965) measured contrast thresholds for sinusoidal grating patterns, grating contrast sensitivity functions have been used to explore normal and abnormal visual systems. Using this simple measure of visual performance, one can integrate results from psychophysical, single-unit recordings and evoked potential studies to develop models of pattern identification and detection, particularly at threshold. Contrast functions are not only used in human visual perception, but are applied in many fields utilizing image displays such as computerized tomography or magnetic resonance imaging in radiology (Sharp, 1987).

It is possible to extrapolate an estimate of Snellen acuity from the contrast sensitivity function. Snellen acuity is analogous to the finest resolvable grating (highest spatial frequency) at which the contrast sensitivity (1/threshold) approaches 1.0. However, since contrast sensitivity functions (CSFs) assess performance across a range of pattern sizes, they can often provide more information about the functioning of the visual system than the assessment of acuity alone. Clinically, Snellen acuity and contrast sensitivity measurements represent complementary aspects of visual performance that may be necessary for accurate diagnosis.

Contrast reflects the variation of luminance across a pattern and its background. The perceived brightness of a target depends on the change of luminance around the border of the target (Fig. 4.1). For grating patterns, contrast is often defined as the difference in luminance between the light bars and the dark bars of a grating divided by the sum of these luminances. As the contrast is lowered, it is more difficult to see the pattern (Fig. 4.2). The amount of contrast needed to detect the presence of the pattern may vary from as little as 0.1% contrast to a maximum of 100% contrast. The grating size is quantified in spatial frequency, a measure of the size of the imaged falling on the

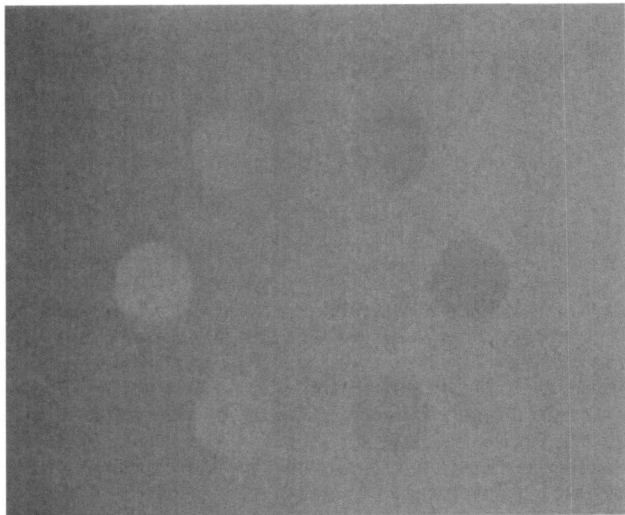

Figure 4.1. Seven equiluminant circles on a background with a linearly varied luminance. The circles on the lighter background appear darker than those on the darker background because of local contrast differences. (Photo courtesy of Robert Shapley, Ph.D.)

Figure 4.2. The contrast is diminished (top to bottom) in a stepwise fashion making, the single spatial frequency sinusoidal gratings progressively more difficult to see. (Photo courtesy of Robert Shapley, Ph.D.)

retina in number of cycles per degree of visual angle. Low spatial frequency patterns are wide bars that are widely spaced, whereas high spatial frequencies are fine bars that are closely spaced (Fig. 4.3).

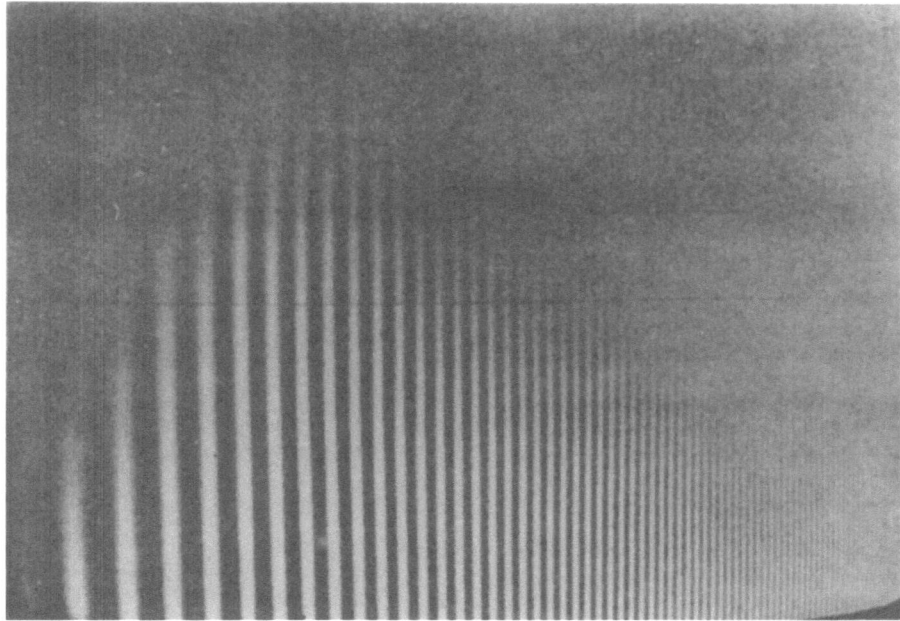

Figure 4.3. The contrast is elevated from top to bottom across a spatial frequency range (low to high, left to right) of sine wave grating. A CSF is immediately apparent. (Photo courtesy of Ivan Bodis-Wollner, M.D.)

Contrast sensitivity functions are derived by measuring the minimum contrast needed to detect the presence of a grating at various spatial frequencies. Contrast sensitivity functions can be obtained using both psychophysical and electrophysiological methods. When CSFs are measured psychophysically, an observer is asked to respond regarding the presence or absence of the pattern. Electrophysiologically, contrast thresholds are typically measured using a zero amplitude criteria (Campbell and Maffei, 1970; Spekrejise et al, 1973).

Contrast sensitivity functions studies in the clinic are most often conducted with gratings whose luminance profile is varied sinusoidally along a single axis, rather than with gratings containing abrupt luminance changes. The rationale for the use of these sinusoidal gratings stems from theories of visual pattern recognition that postulate that the detection occurs via relatively independent channels or mechanisms. A complex scene, therefore, is analyzed into separate components, which are orientation, spatial frequency, and temporal frequency dependent. This is analogous to the type of frequency selectivity performed by the auditory system. The CSF can be thought of as an envelope of separate spatial frequency channels. Sinusoidal gratings are used because of their simplicity in the spatial domain, as opposed to patterns such as checkerboards, which are spatially more complex. Fourier analysis, which is a mathematical description of the spatial components of any pattern stimulus, indicates that checks have pattern components of multiple spatial frequencies along both diagonals, whereas sine wave gratings have only a single spatial frequency along a single axis (DeValois et al, 1979). It is important to note that there are many additional theories of pattern perception.

Recent Studies

Human Psychophysics

The CSF has a characteristic shape (Figs. 4.3 and 4.4) with maximum sensitivity for humans at 3 to 5 c/deg and decreasing sensitivity for both higher and lower spatial frequencies (Campbell and Robson, 1968). The shape of the CSF, however, varies with image movement, mean luminance, and state of retinal luminance adaptation (Kelly, 1977). Contrast sensitivity increases for higher spatial frequencies with a higher background luminance. However, brief exposures of bright light prior to pattern detection elevates the threshold (Crawford, 1947; Tolhurst, 1975). Image stabilization by elimination of eye movements causes low spatial frequency gratings, which were initially seen, to disappear. Increasing eye movement oscillations improves low spatial frequency and diminishes high spatial frequency thresholds. Contrast sensitivity for low spatial frequencies (below 1 c/deg) is improved when the bars of the grating are reversed in time (temporal modulation) at moderate rates (maximally at 10 Hz), whereas sensitivity to high spatial frequencies is impaired under these conditions. On the other hand, there is no attenuation of sensitivity for high spatial frequency gratings at low rates of reversal (Tolhurst, 1973). The CSF obtained with drifting gratings differs from the

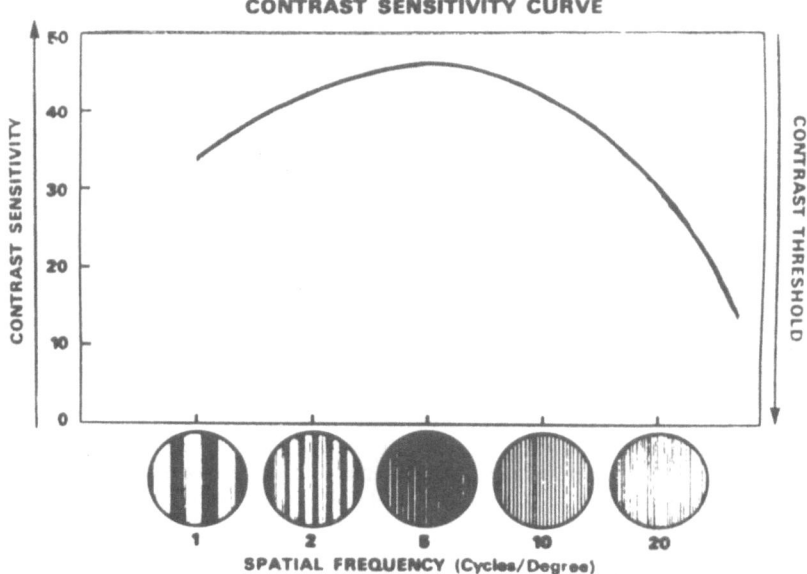

Figure 4.4. A normal CSF plot. As contrast sensitivity increases, less contrast is need to detect the pattern. The peak sensitivity occurs between 3 and 5 c/deg.

CSF obtained with reversing grating, peaking at 12 c/deg (Tolhurst, 1973; Robson, 1966). The sensitivity for higher spatial frequencies is less than that for lower spatial frequencies (0.5 to 1 c/deg) regardless of the temporal frequency (Robson, 1966).

Prior exposure to a grating pattern of a given spatial frequency (Stromeyer et al, 1982; Stecher et al, 1973) and orientation (Blakemore and Campbell, 1969) will cause an elevation of the contrast threshold for that spatial frequency and orientation (spatial adaptation). When only one eye is adapted, this effect transfers to the contralateral eye (interocular transfer), suggesting the involvement of neurons receiving binocular input that are spatial frequency and orientation specific (Blakemore and Campbell, 1969). This adaptation is greatest in the retina closest to the area of the retina exposed to the stimulus (Perizonius et al, 1985). Adaptation occurs immediately upon exposure, even with low contrast adapting patterns, suggesting an active cortical mechanism, such as lateral inhibition, is operational (Dealy and Tolhurst, 1974) rather than a fatigue phenomenon (Swift and Smith 1982). Another perceptual phenomenon, masking, results in reduced visibility of a test pattern when a second pattern (the mask) is presented prior to or simultaneously with the test stimulus. Contrast thresholds are less affected if the masking grating differs from the test grating by more than two octaves (doubling) in spatial frequency.

Contrast detection studies have helped elucidate the mechanisms the human visual system uses in processing spatial patterns (Thomas, 1986; Graham, 1985). Models for pattern detection have been proposed where pattern recognition is performed by channels specific for orientation and spatial frequency (Petersik et al, 1981). A channel may be sensitive over a limited spatial frequency range, such as 1 octave (a factor of 2) above and below the peak spatial frequency. These channels are parallel and probably independent (Stromeyer et al, 1982; Stromeyer and Klein, 1975; Julez and Schumer, 1981). However, not all investigators accept this hypothesis (Henning et al, 1975). Selected mechanisms such as line and edge detection may also be operational (Kulikowski and King-Smith, 1973; Van der Wildt and Waarts, 1983; Shapley and Tolhurst, 1973). The channels may interact and each channel may demonstrate inhibition (Campbell et al, 1969) and/or summation of the responses between them (Jamar and Koenderink, 1985; Kramer et al, 1985). Nonlinearities in this summation may occur (Brogan, 1985; Wilson and Bergen, 1979).

Channels may also exhibit temporal frequency properties (Kulikowski and Tolhurst, 1973). Transient detection occurs mainly for pattern onsets and offsets for low and middle spatial frequency patterns. Sustained detection, over the whole duration of the stimulus cycle, occurs for middle and high spatial frequency patterns. Both spatial frequency (Rovamo and Virsu, 1979) and temporal frequency (Virsu et al, 1982) modulated CSF's are similar at different visual field locations when the equivalent cortical representations are calculated for each by accounting for cortical magnification factors. However, some authors suggest that the central field may be the most important area for determining contrast sensitivity, either for high spatial frequencies or for the whole spatial frequency range, depending on the temporal frequency of the stimulus (Kelly, 1978; Higgins, et al., 1983).

Animal Physiology

Neurophysiological studies of contrast function of single cells in cat and monkey can be used to test models of human pattern perception. Complex pattern analysis begins in the retina, where receptive field organization depends on the relative amounts of luminance-related excitation and inhibition and the temporal interactions between the two. Our understanding of spatial analysis was furthered by the discovery of brisk-sustained linear (X ganglion cells) and brisk-transient nonlinear (Y ganglion cells) responses in the retina to reversing contrast gratings (Enroth-Cugell and Shapley, 1973).

It was suggested that Y cells were motion detectors with nonlinear response functions and that X cells were pattern detectors with linear response functions. An analogous situation has been found in human psychophysics. High-resolution pattern detection is best for stationary or low temporal frequency-modulated gratings. Motion detection is superior forlow spatial frequency but higher temporal frequency gratings (King-Smith and Kulikowski, 1975). In the lateral geniculate, parvocellular layer cells (which may be X cells) are less sensitive to low contrast pattern stimuli, and magnocellular layer cells (which may be Y cells) are more sensitive at lower contrast levels (Shapley and Victor, 1978; Burbeck and Kelly, 1981). The X and Y visual subsystem pathways, at all levels to the visual cortex, may be parallel and subserve different processes (Kaplan and Shapley, 1982). However, not all investigators agree with this classification of distinct visual subsystems, particularly when applied to humans (Lennie, 1980a; 1980b).

Although in man sustained and transient responses have been recorded from retinal ganglion cells, the other physiological and anatomical features of retinal ganglion cells do not fit well into this X and Y classification system. Therefore it is probably more appropriate to categorize human retinal ganglion cells as either magnocellular retinal ganglion cells (M cells) or parvocellular retinal ganglion cells (P cells). The former project to layers 1 and 2 of the lateral geniculate nucleus and the latter to layers 3 through 6. This morphological distinction has been demonstrated in monkey (Leventhal et al., 1981) where the segregation has been shown to continue into the cortex. The magnocellular layer projects to 4C-alpha, which eventually projects to the middle temporal cortical area MT (Zeki, 1969). The parvocellular layer projects to 4C beta of area 17 and then to the pale stripe region of area 18 and finally to areas B3 and B4. The M cell and P cell systems can also be distinguished physiologically. The P cells are characterized by color-opponency, low contrast sensitivity, and high spatial resolution. The M cell system is characterized by absence of color vision, high contrast sensitivity, low spatial resolution, fast temporal resolution, and sensitivity to stereoscopic depth (Livingstone and Hubel, 1987).

There is increased selectivity for spatial frequency moving centrally from the retina to the lateral geniculate to the cortex. Macaque monkey lateral geniculate cells (DeValois et al, 1966) are broadly tuned (responsive over a wide range of spatial frequencies) for spatial frequency whereas the cortical cells are more narrowly tuned. Cortical spatial frequency selectivity is partially independent of orientation - - some cells have narrow spatial frequency (Maffei and Fiorentini, 1973) but broad orientation tuning functions. About 25% of the cortical cells are narrowly tuned for both spatial frequency (0.7 to 1.2 octaves) and orientation (8 degrees to 25 degrees). Cortical cells in the cat demonstrate adaptation to specific spatial frequency gratings (Maffei et al, 1974) and may be organized into functional (Maffei and Fiorentini, 1977) and anatomical (Siliverman et al, 1981; Tootel et al, 1983) columns with a preferred spatial frequency in area 17. A striatal neuron is more sensitive to a sine-wave grating at its optimal spatial frequency grating than to a square-wave bar of any width (Albrecht et al, 1980). Depending on the techniques used, the response of striate neurons increases in a relatively linear fashion over the first 0.5 to 1.0 log units of contrast with a logarithmic change in contrast (Maffei and Fiorentini, 1973; Albrecht and Hamilton, 1982). Neurons of the striate cortex in cats and monkeys also respond selectively to orientation (Hubel and Wiesel, 1968) and are organized into a similar functional columnar architecture (Hubel and Wiesel, 1974; Hubel et al, 1977; Hubel et al, 1978). Orientation and spatial selectivity of cat striate neurons are constant over a large range of contrast changes (Skottun et al, 1987; Sclar and Freeman, 1982). However, in the visual cortex, contrast adaptation, or gain changes, can occur as a function of the mean adapting contrast (Ohzawa et al, 1985). Both adaptation and gain alterations can also be demonstrated to a lesser degree in the lateral geniculate and retina (Shapley and Victor, 1979; Shapley and Victor, 1980). Visual evoked potential studies in the cat have also suggested that spatial adaptation in the cortex seems to be modulated by active inhibitory interactions rather than a fatigue-related process (Bonds, 1984).

Contrast Function Development/Amblyopia/Binocularity

Contrast thresholds have been measured in infants, using a preferential-looking paradigm (Atkinson et al, 1977a). Results from these experiments indicate that contrast sensitivity in infants improves with development throughout the first several years. Infants from 1 to 3 months of age show greater sensitivity for drifting gratings (3 Hz) than stationary gratings (Atkinson et al, 1977b). Narrow-band spatial frequency channels may develop by 12 weeks of age (Banks et al, 1985; Stephens and Banks, 1985). Evoked potential methods demonstrate increased contrast sensitivity for middle and high spatial frequencies in infants over the period of 1 to 6 months (Harris et al, 1976; Pirchio et al, 1978). Thereafter, a small gradual improvement in contrast sensitivity occurs from 2 to 8 years of age (Bradley and Freeman, 1982).

In normal adult observers, binocular contrast thresholds are lower than monocular thresholds (Campbell and Green, 1965). The increased binocular performance is attributed to neural summation between the two eyes because it is greater than the improvement expected on the basis of probability summation, the statistical improvement based on allowing the observer two chances to detect (Blake and Fox, 1973). Binocular summation is maximum when the gratings to each eye are in phase, both spatially (Legge, 1984) and temporally (Westendorf and Fox, 1977). This enhanced sensitivity for binocular targets occurs in infants between 3 and 7 months of age (Teller and Movshon, 1986).

Conditions that interfere with the development of normal binocular vision (e.g., strabismic or anisometropic amblyopia) can produce changes in the CSF. Amblyopia causes impairments in the CSF of the amblyopic eye in both strabismic (Gstalder and Green, 1971; Levi and Harwerth, 1977) and anisometropic individuals (Bradley and Freeman, 1981). In anisometropic amblyopia, this effect is particularly pronounced for high spatial frequency gratings (Bradley and Freeman, 1981). In addition, these observers show little, if any, improvement in the CSF's during binocular viewing (Levi et al, 1979). For anisometropes, those spatial frequencies where the interocular contrast sensitivity differences are greatest are also the spatial frequencies with the most reduced binocular summation (Holopigian et al, 1986). Both anisometropic and strabismic amblyopia produce deficits in temporal frequency processing (Wesson and Loop, 1982). Stabilizing the retinal image (i.e., eliminating the effects of unsteady fixation) does not improve spatial contrast thresholds in an amblyopic eye (Higgins et al, 1982). Normal-vision subjects with induced retinal image motion have reduced sensitivity to high spatial frequencies and enhanced responses to the motion of low spatial frequency gratings. Patients with nystagmus behave in a similar fashion (Dickinson and Abadi, 1985).

Contrast sensitivity diminishes linearly with a decrease in the acuity of the amblyopic eye in humans (Rogers et al, 1987) and monkeys (Smith, et al., 1985). Similarly, astigmatic eyes, which show orientation-specific reduction in acuity at the defocussed meridian (meridional amblyopia), have abnormal CSF even with optical correction (Freeman and Thibos, 1975). Forced preferential-looking techniques have demonstrated similar results in monkeys (Boothe and Teller, 1982). Occlusion therapy will improve contrast sensitivity in the amblyopic eye, particularly at the middle spatial frequencies. Occluding a normal eye for 2 weeks will decrease contrast sensitivity, particularly at middle spatial frequencies, without any changes in acuity (Koskela, 1986).

Optical Factors

Optical, rather than neural, factors may cause abnormalities in CSFs. Contrast sensitivity functions should only be performed when the refractive is corrected. However, the magnification effect of aphakic spectacles decreases the spatial frequency of a grating pattern so the peak of that the CSF is shifted towards the high spatial frequencies. The minification effect of high minus spectacles shifts the peak of the CSF toward the lower spatial frequencies (Enoch et al, 1979a,b). These apparent alterations can be prevented by using a contact lens for CSF determinations in patients with high refractive errors. However, contact lens themselves can induce CSF changes; wearing soft contact lenses for up to 2 weeks, for example, reduces sensitivity (Mitra and Lamberts, 1981; Applegate and Massof, 1975), particularly for high spatial frequencies (Kirkpatrick and Roggenkamp, 1985). Loss of contrast sensitivity also occurs with contact lens induced corneal distortion or with any condition that causes corneal disturbance (Hess and Carney, 1979).

Media opacities, such as cataracts (Skalka, 1981; Owsley et al, 1985), account for part of the middle and high spatial frequency falloff in contrast sensitivity noted with aging, despite the maintenance of 20/20 Snellen acuity. However, diminished retinal illuminance from media opacities is not the sole cause of the reported contrast abnormalities for low spatial frequencies (Sekuler et al, 1980; Skalka, 1980) or middle and high spatial frequencies losses in the elderly (Derefeldt et al, 1979; Owsley et al, 1983). Additionally, adults over the age of 60 do not demonstrate the same motion-induced enhancement of contrast sensitivity for drifting low spatial frequency gratings that younger adults exhibit. This represents a defect in the temporal modulation of vision that cannot be attributed to media opacities.

Ocular Hypertension/Glaucoma

Arden and Jacobson (1978) first demonstrated the utility of contrast gratings for the early detection of glaucoma using grating plates. Contrast losses occur across all spatial frequencies in this disease. Ocular hypertensives with normal fields (Octopus program 33) may demonstrate elevated contrast thresholds (Atkin et al, 1979; Ross et al, 1985). Low and middle spatial frequency contrast deficits have been described with ocular hypertension (Kayazawa et al, 1984). Contrast thresholds may be elevated in family members of patients with glaucoma, even if they are normotensive (Hitchings et al, 1981). The use of miotic drops and concomitant ocular pathology (such as cataracts) in glaucoma patients make the CSF (as well as other subjective visual testing) difficult to compare among patients and even in the single patient over time. However, it remains particularly useful in the ocular hypertensive or in early glaucoma when other ocular pathology is absent.

Retinal Disorders

Many retinal disorders perturb the CSF (Wolkstein et al, 1980). Macular diseases, such as central serous choroidopathy and macular degeneration, elevate the low and middle spatial frequency contrast thresholds when there is relative preservation of acuity (Sjöstrand and Frisén, 1977). As the acuity diminishes, all spatial frequencies, including the high spatial frequencies, demonstrate contrast deficits (Loshin and White, 1984). Retinitis pigmentosa generally depresses the whole CSF in patients with central and peripheral loss, but patients with only ring scotomas may have a normal CSF (Hyvarinen et al, 1981). Diabetic retinopathy causes abnormal CSFs, but in some diabetics without retinopathy, elevated contrast thresholds are also found (Yamazaki et al, 1982).

Optic Neuropathy

Nonselective contrast losses occur with diseases that affect the optic nerves, chiasm, and optic tract. The papilledema of pseudotumor cerebri causes contrast dysfunction that resolves as the disc appearance normalizes (Wall, 1986). Compressive lesions of the anterior visual pathway elevates contrast thresholds prior to acuity, color vision, or visual field loss (Kupersmith et al, 1982a). Except for optic neuritis or multiple sclerosis, contrast deficits are nonselective.

Optic Neuritis/Multiple Sclerosis

Primary demyelinating disease, multiple sclerosis (MS), can cause lesions anywhere in the white matter pathways sensory visual system from the optic nerve to visual cortex. Contrast thresholds for all spatial frequencies are elevated in eyes with acute optic neuritis. Once the neuritis resolves, contrast losses may remain generalized or affect only the low or middle spatial frequencies (Zimmern et al, 1979). The "unaffected" second eye will often demonstrate contrast losses, even if the patient has no other signs of MS (Arden and Gocukogiu, 1978). Patients with MS and no definitive history of optic neuritis can also have elevated contrast thresholds (Kupersmith et al, 1983). Some of these patients have selective losses for middle spatial frequencies (Regan et al, 1977).

In some cases of MS, contrast losses are also orientation selective for one or both eyes (Regan et al, 1980). In other patients, the threshold elevation may be measured at all spatial frequencies but for only one orientation (Kupersmith et al, 1984). Orientation-specific deficits suggest the presence of plaques in the visual cortex and that the cause is not solely in the optic nerve. Contrast sensitivity deficits may also vary with the temporal frequency of the stimulus in patients with optic neuritis. Changing the temporal frequency from 1 to 30 Hz has no appreciable effect on the contrast thresholds for 4 c/deg gratings; but higher temporal frequencies seem to decrease the deficit for a 0.5 c/deg grating (Hess and Plant, 1983).

Cerebral Lesion

Bodis-Wollner first described contrast losses in patients with cerebral lesions with normal ocular examinations findings and visual fields, and with a complaint of blurred vision (Bodis-Wollner and Diamond, 1976). In some patients, contrast sensitivity was reduced uniformly, whereas other patients showed losses specific for high, middle, or low spatial frequencies. Patients with Alzheimer's disease may have elevated contrast thresholds for all spatial frequencies (Schlotterer et al, 1983; Nissen et al, 1985). Visual system involvement in Parkinson's disease can be demonstrated by contrast sensitivity defects that are nonselective for spatial frequency (Kupersmith et al, 1982b). Contrast threshold elevation also occurs in normals when dopaminergic transmission is blocked by dopaminergic antagonist drugs (Domenici et al, 1985). Orientation-specific losses seem to reflect cortical dysfunction in Parkinson's patients without dementia (Regan and Maxner, 1987).

Technical Aspects

Though contrast sensitivity testing gives a more complete analysis of spatial-pattern vision than Snellen acuity, the numerous methods and variability of CSFs among subjects can frustrate the clinician. Thresholds vary with criteria used, such as movement or flicker (for moving gratings) detection, versus pattern appears or disappearance. Movement criteria gives lower thresholds for lower spatial frequencies. Also, contrast thresholds are often higher when the contrast is raised from subthreshold until the pattern appears (ascending limit), as compared with the threshold obtained starting with easily seen gratings (suprathreshold) and the contrast is lowered until the pattern disappears (descending limit). Besides the ascending and descending limits method (where either the subject or the tester adjusts the contrast), a more difficult but typically more precise technique a forced choice approach is commonly used. The observer is asked to identify the pattern on one or more visual displays. The method of constant stimuli records the number or percentage of correct responses for a fixed spatial frequency over a range of spatial frequencies. Preferential-looking techniques are used to study nonverbal subjects such as infants. When presented two visual displays, it is assumed that the subject will look at the more "interesting" visual stimulus, when one contains enough contrast for a pattern to be seen (Banks and Ginsburg, 1985). When the method of constant stimuli is used, the observer is shown gratings of different contrast, varying from subthreshold to easily visible, in a random order. The number of times the subject sees the pattern is recorded for each contrast level; the threshold is the contrast that gives a pattern detection response in at least 50% of the trials. In the staircase method, the contrast is decreased until the pattern is invisible; contrast is then raised until the pattern is seen. This process is repeated until a predetermined number of staircase reversals occurs. The threshold is defined as the average contrast of these staircase reversals.

Different methods of producing sine-wave gratings also contribute to the lack of uniformity of CSF data. Electronically generated sine-wave gratings are used for most experimental studies and give the greatest flexibility for changing the spatial and temporal parameters of the test patterns. Oscilloscope screens are excellent for displaying high spatial frequency gratings, but the displays are usually too small to accommodate sufficient numbers of cycles of low spatial frequency gratings. In contrast, television displays are larger and brighter. However, it is difficult to generate high spatial frequency, drifting or oblique gratings, and a distracting flicker of the display may occur. The luminance of the cathode ray tube screens can vary from below 25 cd/M^2 to 1000 candelas/meter^2. Extremes of luminance of a test screen can change the contrast thresholds (Weber's law). The orientation of the gratings can be rotated with some but not all pattern generators.

Normal subjects will have thresholds that are lower for horizontal and vertical than for obliquely, oriented gratings (Berkley et al, 1975; Camisa et al, 1977). Changing the orientation between successive contrast determinations can minimize the spatial adaptation-induced threshold elevation that results from retesting with a similar spatial frequency and orientation grating.

Gratings may be static, counter-reversed, or drifted perpendicularly to the axis of the stripes. Thresholds are higher for temporally modulated gratings than for static gratings when high spatial frequency gratings are studied. Conversely, thresholds for temporally modulated gratings, particularly at high temporal frequencies, are superior for low spatial frequencies than when a static pattern is used. This peak spatial sensitivity also shifts with changes in the temporal frequency.

Contrast sensitivity charts are commonly used in clinical practice. The Arden plates and the Vistec charts (Arden, 1978; Ginsburg, 1984) are two photographic displays in widespread application. Recently, low contrast Snellen letter charts have been introduced and can reveal contrast losses similar to those demonstrated by sine-wave gratings (Regan and Neima, 1983). These chart displays are limited by a lack of flexibility and temporal and orientation factors are not considered.

Future of the Test

Investigators are currently attempting to find rates of temporal modulation that can discriminate between the M cell and P cell functions. The hope is that specific disease entities may be characterized by the predominant loss of one ganglion cell type. For example, it has been proposed that glaucoma is predominantly an M cell retinal ganglion cell disorder.

Automated perimetry using contrast sensitivity targets is currently being investigated. Preliminary studies suggest that contrast sensitivity is more sensitive than differential light threshold perimetry for visual field defect detection (Neima et al, 1984). Novel modes of stimulus presentation may enhance contrast sensitivity testing. An example of this is contrast targets generated by a variable contrast laser interferometer.

Summary

Contrast sensitivity testing has proved effective in uncovering hidden visual loss that would not be revealed by other measures of visual performance. Contrast losses that are selective for spatial frequency or orientation or temporal frequency imply dysfunction of specific neuronal populations or visual subsystems. When properly performed on attentive subjects, the findings are reliable and consistent, yielding pathology more than other clinical visual tests. The results of contrast threshold determinations across the spatial/temporal domain are useful in developing hypotheses of pattern discrimination and spatial analysis.

References

Albrecht DG, Hamilton DB. Striate cortex of monkey and cat: Contrast response function. J Neurophysiol 1982;48:217-37.

Albrecht DG, DeValois RL, Thorell LG. Visual cortex neurons: Are bars or gratings the optimal stimuli? Science 1980;207:88-90.

Applegate RA, Massof RW. Changes in the contrast sensitivity function induced by contact lens wear. Am J Optom Physiol Opti 1975;52:840-46.

Arden GB, Gocukogiu AG. Grating test of contrast sensitivity in patients with retrobulbar neuritis. Arch Ophthalmol 1978;96:1626-29.

Arden GB, Jacobson JJ. A simple grating test for contrast sensitivity: Preliminary results indicate value in screening glaucoma. Invest Ophthalmol Vis Sci 1978;17:2332.

Arden GB. The importance of measuring contrast sensitivity in cases of visual disturbance. Br J Ophthalmol 1978;62:198-9.

Atkin A, Bodis Wollner I, Wolkstein M, et al. Abnormalities of central contrast sensitivity in glaucoma. Am J Ophthalmol 1979;88:205-11.

Atkinson J, Braddick O, Moar K. Contrast sensitivity of the human infant for moving and static patterns. Vis Res 1977a;17:1045-47.

Atkinson J, Braddick O, Moar K. Development of contrast sensitivity over the first 3 months of life in the human infant. Vis Res 1977a;17:1037-44.

Banks MS, Ginsburg AP. Infant visual preferences: A review and new theoretical treatment. Adv Child Dev Behavi 1985;19:207-46.

Banks MS, Stephens BR, Hartmann EE. The development of basic mechanisms of pattern vision: Spatial frequency channels. J Exp Child Psychol 1985;40:501-27.

Berkley MA, Kitterle F, Watkins DW. Grating visibility as a function of orientation and retinal eccentricity. Vision Res 1975;15:239-44.

Blake, R., Fox, R. The psychophysical inquiry into binocular summation. Percept Psychophys 1973:14:161-85.

Blakemore C, Campbell RW. On the existence of neurones in the human visual system selectively sensitive to the orientation and rise of retinal images. J Physiol 1969;203:237-60.

Bodis-Wollner I, Diamond SP. The measurement of spatial contrast sensitivity in cases of blurred vision associated with cerebral lesions. Brain 1976;99:695-710.

Bonds AB. Spatial adaptation of the cortical visual evoked potential of the cat. Invest Ophthalmol Vis Sci 1984;25:640-6.

Boothe RG, Teller DY. Meridional variations in acuity and CSF's in monkeys (Macacca nemestrina) reared with externally applied astigmatism. Vis Res 1982;22:801-10.

Bradley A, Freeman RD. Contrast sensitivity in anisometropic amblyopia. Invest Ophthalmol Vis Sci 1981;21:467-76.

Bradley A, Freeman RD. Contrast sensitivity in children. Vis Res 1982;22:953-59.

Brogan D. Spatial frequency range in the detection process1. Narrow bars. Ophthalmic Physiol Opt 1985;5:125-35.

Burbeck CA, Kelly D. Contrast gain measurements and transient/sustained dichotomy. J Opt Soc Am 1981;71:1335-42.

Camisa JM, Blake R, Lema S. The effects of temporal modulation on the oblique effect in humans. Perception 1977;6:165-71.

Campbell FW, Green DG. Optical and retinal factors affecting visual resolution. J Physiol 1965;181:576-92.

Campbell FW, Maffei L. Electrophysiological evidence for the existence of orientation and size detectors in the human visual system. J Physiol 1970;207:635-52.

Campbell FW, Robson JG. Application of Fourier analysis to the visibility of gratings. J Physiol 1968;197:551-66.

Campbell FW, Carpenter RHS, Levinson JZ. Visibility of aperiodic patterns compared with that of sinusoidal gratings. J Physiol 1969;204:283-98.

Crawford BH. Visual adaptation relating to brief conditioning flashes. Proc R Soc 1947;134:283-302.

Dealy RS, Tolhurst DJ. Is spatial adaptation an aftereffect of prolonged inhibition? J Physiol 1974;241:261-70.

Derefeldt G, Lennerstrand G, Lundh B. Age variations in normal human contrast sensitivity. Acta Ophthalmol 1979;57:679.

DeValois K, DeValois R, Yund E. Responses of striate cortex cells to grating and checker board patterns. J Physiol 1979;291:483-505.

DeValois RL, Abramov I, Jacobs GH. Analysis of response patterns of LGN cells. J Opt Soc Am 1966;56:966-77.

Dickinson CM, Abadi RV. The influence of nystagmoid oscillation on contrast sensitivity in normal observers. Vis Res 1985;25:1089-96.

Domenici L, Trimarchi C, Piccolino M, et al. Dopaminergic drugs improve human visual contrast sensitivity. Human Neurobiol 1985;4:195-7.

Enoch JM, Ohzu H, Motokazu I. Contrast (modulation) sensitivity functions measured in patients with high refractive error with emphasis on aphakia: I. Theoretical considerations. Doc Ophthalmol 1979a;47:139-45.

Enoch JM, Shinichi Y, Namba A. Contrast (modulation) sensitivity functions measured in patients with high refractive error with emphasis on aphakia: II. Determinations on patients. Doc Ophthalmol 1979b;47:147-62.

Enroth-Cugell C, Shapley RM. Adaptation and dynamics of cat retinal ganglion cells. J Physiol 1973;233:271-309.

Freeman RD, Thibos LN. Contrast sensitivity in humans with abnormal visual experience. J Physiol 1975;247:687-710.

Ginsburg AP. A new contrast sensitivity vision test chart. Am J Optom Physiol Opt 1984;61:463-7.

Graham N. Detection and identification of near threshold visual patterns. J Opt Soc Am 1985;2:1468-82.

Gstalder RJ, Green DG. Laser interferometric acuity in amblyopia. J Pediatr Ophthalmol 1971;8:251-65.

Harris L, Atkinson J, Braddick O. Visual contrast sensitivity of a 6 month old infant measured by the evoked potential. Nature 1976;264:570-1.

Henning GB, Hertz BG, Broadbent DE. Some experiments bearing on the hypothesis that the visual system analyses spatial patterns in independent bands of spatial frequency. Vis Res 1975;15:887-97.

Hess RF, Carney LG. Vision through and abnormal cornea: A pilot study of the relationship between visual loss from corneal distortion, corneal edema, keratoconus, and some allied corneal pathology. Invest Ophthalmol Vis Sci 1979;18:476-83.

Hess RF, Plant GT. The effect of temporal frequency variation on threshold contrast sensitivity deficits inoptic neuritis. J Neurol Neurosurg Psychiatr 1983;46:322-30.

Higgins KE, Caruso RC, Coletta NJ, de Monasterio FM. Effect of artificial central scotoma on the spatial contrast sensitivity of normal subjects. Invest Ophthalmol Vis Sci 1983;24:1131-38.

Higgins KE, Daugman JG, Mansfield RJW. Amblyopic contrast sensitivity: insensitivity to unsteady fixation. Invest Ophthalmol Vis Sci 1982;23: 113-20.

Hitchings RA, Powell DJ, Arden GB, Carter RM. Contrast sensitivity gratings in glaucoma family screening. Br J Ophthalmol 1981;65:515-17.

Holopigian K, Blake R, Greenwald MJ. Selective losses in binocular vision in anisometropic amblyopes. Vis Res 1986;26:621-30.

Hubel DH, Wiesel TN. Receptive fields and functional architecture of monkey striate cortex. J Physiol 1968;195:215-43.

Hubel DH, Wiesel TN. Sequence regularity and geometry of orientation columns in the monkey striate cortex. J Comp Neurol 1974;158:267-93.

Hubel DH, Wiesel TN, Stryker MP. Anatomical demonstration of orientation columns in macaque monkey. J Comp Neurol 1978;177:361-80.

Hubel DH, Wiesel TN, Stryker MP. Orientation columns in macaque monkey visual cortex demonstrated by the 2 deoxyglucose autoradiographic technique. Nature 1977;269:328-30.

Hyvarinen L, Rovamo J, Laurinen P, et al. Contrast sensitivity function in evaluation of visual impairment due to retinitis pigmentosa. Acta Ophthalmol 1981;59:763-73.

Jamar JHT, Koenderink JJ. Contrast detection and detection of contrast modulation for noise gratings. Vis Res 1985;25:511-21.

Julez B, Schumer RA. Early visual perception. Ann Rev Psycholol 1981;32:575-627.

Kaplan E, Shapley R. X and Y cells in the lateral geniculate nucleus of macaque monkeys. J Physiol 1982;330:125-43.

Kayazawa F, Nishimura K, Tanage T, et al. Contrast sensitivity function in primary open angle glaucoma. Glaucoma 1984;6:13-6.

Kelly DH. Photopic contrast sensitivity without foveal vision. Opt Let 1978;2:7-9.

Kelly DH. Visual contrast sensitivity. Opti Acta 1977;24:107-29.

King-Smith PE, Kulikowski JJ. Pattern and flicker detection analyzed by subthreshold summation. Physiol 1975;249:519-48.

Kirkpatrick DL, Roggenkamp JR. Effects of soft contact lenses on contrast sensitivity. Am J Optom Physiol Opt 1985;62:407-12.

Koskela PU. Contrast sensitivity in amblyopia II. Changes during pleoptic treatment. Acta Ophthalmol 1986;64:563-69.

Kramer P, Graham N, Yager D. Simultaneous measurement of spatial frequency summation and uncertainty effects. J Opt Soc Am 1985;2:1533-42.

Kulikowski JJ, King-Smith PE. Spatial arrangement of line, edge and grating detectors revealed by subthreshold summation. Vis Res 1973;13:1455-78.

Kulikowski JJ, Tolhurst DJ. Psychophysical evidence for sustained and transient detectors in human vision. J Physiol 1973;232:149-62.

Kupersmith M, Siegel I, Carr R. Subtle disturbances of vision with compressive lesions of the anterior visual pathway measured by contrast sensitivity. Ophthalmology 1982a;82:68-72.

Kupersmith M, Siegel I, Shakin E, Lieberman A. Visual system dysfunction in Parkinson's disease. Arch Neurol 1982b;39:284-86.

Kupersmith MJ, Nelson JI, Seiple WH, Carr RE, Weiss PA. The 20/20 eye in multiple sclerosis. Neurology 1983;33:101-2.

Kupersmith MJ, Seiple WH, Nelson JI, Carr, RE. Contrast sensitivity loss in multiple sclerosis. Selectivity by eye, orientation, and spatial frequency measured with the evoked potential. Invest Ophthalmol Vis Sci 1984;25:632-9.

Legge GE. Binocular contrast summation I. Detection and discrimination. Vis Res 1984;24:373-83.

Lennie P. Perceptual signs of parallel pathways. Philos Trans R Soc Lond Biol 1980a;290:pp. 23-7.

Lennie P. Parallel visual pathways: a review. Vis Res 1980b;20:561-94.

Leventhal AG, Rodieck RW, Dreher B. Retinal ganglion cell classes in the old world monkey. Morphology and central projections. Science 1981;213:1139-42.

Levi, D. M., Harwerth, R.S. Spatiotemporal interactions in anisometropic and strabismic amblyopia. Invest Ophthalmol Vis Sci 1977;16:90-5.

Levi DM, Harwerth RS, Smith EL. III. Humans deprived of normal binocular vision have binocular interactions tuned to size and orientation. Science 1979;206:852-54.

Livingstone MS, Hubel DH. Psychophysical evidence for separate channels for the perception of form, color, movement and depth. J Neurosci 1987;7:3416-68.

Loshin DS, White J. Contrast sensitivity. The visual rehabilitation of the patient with macular degeneration. Arch Ophthalmol 1984;102:1303-6.

Maffei L, Fiorentini A. Spatial frequency rows in the striate visual cortex. Vis Res 1977;17:357-61.

Maffei L, Fiorentini A. The visual cortex as a spatial frequency analyzer. Vis Res 1973;13:1255-67.

Maffei L, Fiorentini A, Bisti S. Neural correlate of perceptual adaptation to grating. Science 1974;182:1036-38.

Mitra S, Lamberts DW. Contrast sensitivity in soft lens wearers. Contact Intraocul Lens Med J 1981;7:315-22.

Neima D, LeBlanc R, Regan D. Visual field defects in ocular hypertension and glaucoma. Arch Ophthalmol 1984;102:1042-5.

Nissen MJ, Corkin S, Buonanno FS, Growdon J, Wray S, Bauer J. Spatial vision in Alzheimer's disease. Arch Neurol 1985;42:667-71.

Ohzawa I, Sclar G, Freeman RD. Contrast gain control in the cat visual cortex. Nature 1982;298:266-8.

Ohzawa I, Sclar G, Freeman RD. Contrast gain control in the cat's visual system. J Neurophysiol 1985;54:651-67.

Owsley C, Gardner T, Sekuler R, Lieberman H. Role of the crystalline lens in the spatial vision loss of the elderly. Invest Ophthalmol Vis Sci 1985;26:1165-70.

Owsley C, Sekuler R, Siemsen D. Contrast sensitivity throughout adulthood. Vis Res 1983;23:689-99.

Perizonius E, Schill W, Geiger H, Rohler R. Evidence on the local character of spatial frequency channels in the human visual system. Vis Res 1985;25:1233-40.

Petersik JT, Beverley KI, Regan D. Contrast sensitivity of the changing size channel. Vis Res 1981;21:829-32.

Pirchio M, Spinelli D, Fiorentini A, Maffei L. Infant contrast sensitivity evaluated by evoked potentials. Brain Res 1978;141:179-84.

Regan D, Maxner C. Orientation selective visual loss in patients with Parkinson's disease. Brain 1987;110:415-32.

Regan D, Neima D. Low contrast letter charts as a test of visual function. Ophthalmology 1983;90:1192-1200.

Regan D, Silver R, Murray TJ. Visual acuity and contrast sensitivity in multiple sclerosis Hidden visual loss. An auxiliary diagnostic test. Brain 1977;100:563-79.

Regan D, Whitlock JA, Murray TJ, Beverley KI. Orientation specific losses of contrast sensitivity in multiple sclerosis. Invest Ophthalmol Vis Sci 1980;19:324-28.

Robson JG. Spatial and temporal contrast sensitivity functions of the visual system. J Opt Soc Am 1966;56:1141-2.

Rogers GL, Bremer DL, Leguire LE. The contrast sensitivity function and childhood amblyopia. Am J Ophthalmol 1987;104:64-8.

Ross JE, Bron AJ, Reeves BC, Emmerson PG. Detection of optic nerve damage in ocular hypertension. Br J Ophthalmol 1985;69:897-903.

Rovamo J, Virsu V. An estimation and application of the human cortical magnification factor. Exp Brain Res 1979;37:495-10.

Schlotterer G, Moscovitch M, Crapper McLachland D. Visual processing deficits as assessed by spatial frequency contrast sensitivity and backward masking in normal aging and Alzheimer's disease. Brain 1983;107:309-25.

Sclar G, Freeman RD. Orientation selectivity in the cat's striate cortex is invariant with stimulus contrast. Exp Brain Res 1982;46:457-61.

Sekuler R, Hutman LP, Owsley CJ. Human aging and spatial vision. Science 1980;209:1255-6.

Shapley R, Victor JD. The contrast gain control of the cat retina. Vis Res 1979;19:431-4.

Shapley RM, Tolhurst DJ. Edge detectors in the human visual system. J Physiol 1973;229:165-83.

Shapley RM, Victor JD. The effect of contrast on the transfer properties of cat retinal ganglion cells. J Physiol 1978;285:275-98.

Shapley RM, Victor JD: The effect of contrast on the nonlinear response of the Y cell. J Physiol 1980;302:535-47.

Sharp PF. Image perception. IEEE Proc 1987;134:211-24.

Silverman MS, Tootell RBH, DeValois RL. Electrophysiological verification of deoxyglucose spatial frequency columns in cat striate cortex. Soc Neurosci Abstr 1981;111:3-56.

Sjöstrand J, Frisén L. Contrast sensitivity in macular disease. Acta Ophthalmol 1977;55:507-14.

Skalka HW. Arden grating test in evaluating "early" posterior subcapsular cataracts. South Med J 1981;74:1368-70.

Skalka HW. Effect of age on Arden grating acuity. Br J Ophthalmol 1980;64:21-3.

Skottun BC, Bradley A, Sclar G, et al. The effects of contrast on visual orientation and spatial frequency discrimination: A comparison of single cells and behavior. J Neurophysiol 1987;57:773-86.

Smith EL, Harwerth RS, Crawford MLJ. Spatial contrast sensitivity deficits in monkeys produced by optically induced anisometropia. Invest Ophthalmol Vis Sci 1985;26:330-42.

Spekrejise H, Vand Der Tweel LH, Zundema T. Contrast evoked responses in man. Vis Res 1973;13:1577-1601.

Stecher S, Sigel C, Lange RV. Spatial frequency channels inhuman vision and the threshold for adaptation. Vis Res 1973;13:1691-1700.

Stephens BR and Banks MS. The development of contrast constancy. J Exp Child Psychol 1985;40:528-47.

Stromeyer CF, Klein S. Evidence against narrow band spatial frequency channels in human vision: The detectability of frequency modulated gratings. Vis Res 1975;15:899-10.

Stromeyer CF, Klein S, Dawson BM, Spillman L. Low spatial frequency channels in human vision: Adaptation and masking. Vis Res 1982;22:225-33.

Swift DJ, Smith RA. An action spectrum for spatial frequency adaptation. Vis Res 1982;22:235-46.

Teller DY, Movshon JA. Visual development. Vis Res 1986;26:1483-1506.

Thomas JP. Spatial vision then and now. Vis Res 1986;26:1523-30.

Tolhurst DJ. Separate channels for the analysis of the shape and the movement of a moving visual stimulus. J Physiol 1973;231:385-402.

Tolhurst DJ. Sustained and transient channels in human vision. Vis Res 1975;15:1151-5.

Tootell RBH, Silverman MS, DeValois RL, Jacobs GH. Functional organization of the second cortical visual areain primates. Science 1983;220:7-37.

Van der Wildt GJ, Waarts RG. Contrast detection and its dependence on the presence of edges and lines in the stimulus field. Vis Res 1983;23:821-30.

Virsu V, Rovamo J, Laurinen P, Nasanen R. Temporal contrast sensitivity and cortical magnification. Vis Res 1982;22:1211-7.

Wall M. Contrast sensitivity testing in pseudotumor cerebri. Ophthalmology 1986;93:4-7.

Wesson MD, Loop MS. Temporal contrast sensitivity in amblyopia. Invest Ophthal Vis Sci 1982;22:98-102.

Westendorf D H, Fox R. Binocular detection of disparate light flashes. Vis Res 1977;17:697-702.

Wilson HR Bergen JR. A four mechanism model for threshold spatial vision. Vis Res 1979;19:19-32.

Wolkstein M, Atkin A, Bodis Wollner I. Contrast sensitivity in retinal disease. Am J Ophthalmol 1980;87:1140-49.

Yamazaki H, AdachiUsami E, Chiba J. Contrast thresholds of diabetic patients determined by VECP and psychophysical measurements. Acta Ophthalmol 1982;60:386-92.

Zeki SM. Representation of central visual fields in prestriate cortex of monkeys. Brain Res 1969;14:271-91.

Zimmern RL, Campbell FW, Wilkinson IMS. Subtle disturbances of vision after optic neuritis elicited by studying contrast sensitivity. J Neurol Neurosurg Psychiatr 1979;42:407-12.

Chapter 5

New Methods in Clinical Electrophysiology

Thomas E. Ogden

Carl J. Bassi

Introduction

The basics of clinical electrophysiology were well established by the 1960s, and standard procedures have changed little since that time. The most important recent innovation has been the advent of the personal computer and the wide availability of new computer-based equipment for use in clinical practice. In keeping with the emphasis of this book on new developments, only brief mention is made of standard use of the electro-oculogram (EOG), electroretinogram (ERG), and visual evoked potential (VEP). The reader is referred to Carr and Siegel (1982) for a review of these topics. This book also contains an extensive bibliography. A number of nonstandard research developments for diagnosis and localization of abnormalities in the visual system using electrophysiology are presented. These are new in the sense that the procedures are not generally used, but each holds promise of a contribution to the clinical practice of ophthalmology. Not all new procedures are described, but rather, for the most part, those with which the authors have had at least minimal experience.

This chapter will explore both standard and nonstandard ways of assessing functional capabilities of the visual system beginning with the retinal pigment epithelium-photoreceptor complex, continuing through the retina, and finally along the higher visual pathways.

Electrophysiologic Tests

EOG

The EOG is an electrical test of the function of the complex of retinal photoreceptors and retinal pigment epithelium (RPE). In the normal eye there is a difference of potential between the cornea and the back of the globe amounting to about 0.01 V. This standing potential is large when the eye is light adapted and is reduced to about half its light-adapted value when the eye is dark adapted. Thus the ratio of light-adapted value to dark-adapted value, the "light/dark ratio," is normally about 2.0. Any disease that affects the health of the RPE-photoreceptor complex over a large area of the retina causes a reduction of the light/dark ratio. A value of 1.6 is considered borderline normal, and a value of 1.5 or less indicates abnormality with a high degree of reliability.

The EOG cannot be recorded directly because an electrode cannot be placed noninvasively behind the eyeball. It can be recorded indirectly, however. This is accomplished by placing recording electrodes at the inner and outer canthi. When the pupil, which has a positive charge, is midway between these two electrodes, no voltage difference is detected between them. When the eye is abducted, the positive cornea is brought closer to the outer electrode, and a voltage difference is recorded with the outer electrode more positive than the inner. The opposite happens when the eye is adducted.

The magnitude of the voltage recorded when the eye moves is proportional to the standing potential as indicated above and varies normally with the state of adaptation of the eye. In practice the eye movement voltage is recorded at intervals over a 30-minute period as the patient fixates alternatively on a pair of fixation lights separated by a visual angle of 30 degrees. During the initial 15 minutes of recording, the eye is dark adapted and the voltage gradually declines. During the second half of the recording the eye is light adapted, and the voltage approximately doubles in amplitude if the eye is normal. The light/dark ratio is calculated by dividing the smallest amplitude observed during dark adaptation into the largest amplitude recorded during light adaptation.

The test is reliable if light adaptation is adequate and the eye movements are reasonably precise and reproducible. The test does not work well in small children because of their short attention span and is not reliable in the presence of any motor problem that interferes with regular, controlled eye movements. It is also unreliable in the presence of any condition that interferes with adequate light adaptation.

Direct Current ERG

The standard EOG is invaluable in the diagnosis of tapetoretinal abnormalities, but it can be difficult to measure in patients with large central scotomas, severely constricted visual fields, or in patients unwilling to elicit standard eye movements. Two tests, the direct current ERG and the eye blink EOG, are potentially useful tests in assessing tapetoretinal function in these patients.

The ERG, as used in clinical practice, is recorded with capacitor-coupled amplifiers to block baseline drift caused by battery potentials of the metallic electrodes. This recording technique is referred to as alternating current (AC), since only signals that change with time are amplified. Unchanging or constant voltage levels are filtered out of AC recordings.

By use of special (direct current) (DC) amplifiers, it is possible to detect voltages that are constant or change only very slowly with time. This recording technique requires the use of nonpolarizable electrodes. These are difficult to use and poorly adapted to use with patients. Hence the DC-ERG, although well known for more than 20 years, has not been used widely for diagnostic electrophysiology.

DuBois-Reymond (1849) was the first to observe the corneofundal potential that causes the cornea to be about 10 mV positive with reference to the posterior pole of the eye. That the corneofundal potential undergoes slow fluctuations in the dark and changes slowly in response to illumination of the retina has been known for more than a century (Kühne and Steiner, 1881).

As noted above, the corneofundal potential is the basis of the EOG (Arden and Barrada, 1962). Interest in use of the EOG as a measure of retinal function is based primarily on identification of the RPE as the generator of a major contribution to the light-sensitive portion of the potential. Noell (1953) associated loss of the corneofundal potential with RPE damage in rabbits poisoned with iodoacetic acid. This association was later confirmed by numerous workers, and the ionic basis of the potential was eventually established in a series of studies done in the laboratories of Roy Steinberg (e.g., Linsenmeier and Steinberg 1987; Miller and Steinberg, 1977a,b). Steinberg (1985) describes three separate RPE cell membrane polarizations in response to light.

Following illumination, there is first hyperpolarization of the RPE apical membrane, peaking at 4 seconds; this is followed by a delayed hyperpolarization of the basal membrane of the RPE cells, peaking 20 seconds after the onset of illumination. This is followed by a slow depolarization that accounts for the light peak of the EOG and occurs at 5 minutes in the cat and at about 10 minutes in man. The first hyperpolarization causes the c-wave of the ERG. The delayed hyperpolarization accounts for the fast oscillation of the EOG.

Few attempts to record DC-ERGs were made prior to the development of improved methods of recording (Knave et al, 1973). Successful recordings were obtained by Dodt (1951), Wirth (1951), Hanitzsch et al (1966), and Heilig et al (1973). With the use of calomel electrodes, Skoog (1974), Skoog and Nilsson (1974), and Nilsson and Skoog (1975) obtained stable recordings showing covariation of the c-wave and standing potential, their relation to stimulus intensity, cyclic variations of these potentials, and the effect of ethyl alcohol on them (Textorius, 1978; Taumer et al 1976a-c).

Experimental studies with perfused mammalian eyes have shown high oxygen dependency of the corneofundal potential and sensitivity to pH changes (Niemeyer, 1983).

There have been few attempts to apply DC recording clinically. Using vacuum electrodes, Taumer et al (1976a-c) recorded well-developed c-waves and showed the light rise of the corneofundal potential (Fig. 5.1). Other workers recorded the DC-ERG from patients with hemeralopia congenita (Heilig et al, 1973), central retinal artery occlusion (Textorius, 1978; Textorius et al 1978), and various anesthetic agents. The DC-ERG has also been used to register changes in the diameter of the pupil.

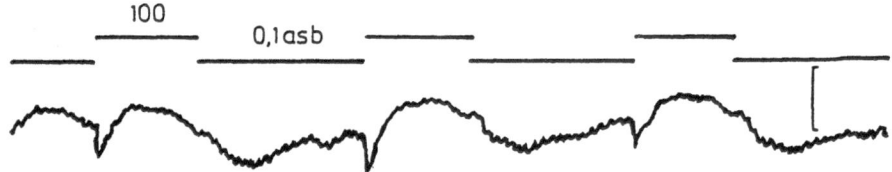

Figure 5.1. Response of retinal potential to light stimuli (100 asb) of 12-s duration recorded by the DC-ERG technique. (redrawn with permission from Taumer et al, 1976a).

In summary, although a great deal is known about the cellular basis of the corneofundal potential and ERG c-wave, their registration presents sufficiently severe technical problems to preclude widespread clinical use. The DC-ERG is a useful research tool and provides valuable information concerning RPE function. With the future development of improved recording procedures, the electrodiagnosis of RPE dysfunction with DC recording will be aided greatly.

Eye-Blink EOG

The eye-blink EOG (Denny and Denny, 1984) is based on the assumption that the most of the potential associated with involuntary eye blinks (Matsuo et al, 1975) is generated by the corneofundal potential.

Comparison of the standard EOG and eye-blink EOG revealed a close match in the responses. There was actually less variability in the eye-blink responses than in the standard responses. However, the specificity and reliability of this test in patients with tapetoretinal disorders are currently untested.

Stress Tests of RPE Function

Whereas the standard EOG measures tapetoretinal function, stress tests (hyperosmolarity, Diamox) may provide specific information about only the RPE.

Standing Potential Hyperosmolarity Test

Yonemura and Kawasaki (1979) have developed a provocative test of the corneofundal potential that probably reflects RPE function independently of photoreceptor function. The EOG amplitude, which reflects the magnitude of the corneofundal potential, is recorded during intravenous injection of a hypertonic solution (14% mannitol, 10% fructose; 1400 mOsm). The effect of the solution is to abolish the light rise and reduce the EOG amplitude to about 75% of the dark trough within about 15 minutes. The effect lasts about 1 hour and is not sensitive to rate of infusion or concentration of solution providing it exceeded 1,140 mOsm and 2.37 mL/kg body weight. The authors report abnormal hyperosmolarity responses in seven of eight eyes with diabetic retinopathy but normal EOGs. The test was also abnormal in five patients with retinitis pigmentosa and in two patients with central retinal artery occlusion in whom the EOG, initially abnormal, had returned to normal. Thus, the hyperosmolarity stress test may be a more sensitive test of presumed RPE function than the EOG alone.

Diamox-Stress Test

Yonemura and Kawasaki (1979) also reported reduction of the corneofundal potential by Diamox. This is probably due to an effect on the RPE since Steinberg and Miller (1973) found that Diamox reduced the isolated trans-RPE potential in the frog retina. Diamox, 500 mg intravenously, lowers the EOG dark trough amplitude by 40%. Unlike the hyperosmolarity test, the Diamox-stress test response was normal in patients with diabetic retinopathy and retinitis pigmentosa but abnormal in patients with pigment epitheliopathy of the posterior pole involving at least 3 disc diameters of retina. The Diamox response is normal in virtually total retinal detachment, indicating its independence of photoreceptor function.

These tests involve little discomfort to the patient but require about 45 minutes to 1 hour of recording time. The Diamox test may be of use in evaluation of subtle RPE defects in the posterior pole in patients whose other electrophysiology test result are normal.

ERG

Continuing further in the visual pathway, the electrical responses of the retina, the ERG, will be discussed. First a brief description of the standard ERG will be presented, followed by newer tests developed to evaluate specific retinal cell types or to test specific retinal areas.

The ERG is a transient voltage evoked in the retina by a flash of light. It is usually recorded from the fully dilated eye, with the active electrode on the cornea against a reference electrode on the conjunctiva (bipolar Burian-Allen electrode), or on the forehead or ear lobe (unipolar recording). The ERG is evoked with a brief, xenon flash to a diffusing screen, a frosted lens, a diffusing bowl, or into a Ping-Pong ball. This diffusing screen effectively illuminates the entire retina in what is referred to as a ganzfeld, "complete field", illumination. This full-field retinal stimulation is essential to ensure equivalent and simultaneous activation of the entire retina. Less than full-field stimulation will evoke mixed responses from fully stimulated retina and retina weakly stimulated by scattered light, and this will produce responses whose waveforms are ambiguous. Also, amplitude measures are valid only under conditions of standard total retinal illumination.

The ERG waveform results from the summation of voltages from two principal sources: (a) receptors and (b) postsynaptic cells, including Müller cells. The receptors act first to generate a cornea-negative wave called the late-receptor potential (Brown and Watanabe, 1962a,b; Brown et al, 1965; Brown, 1968). The late-receptor potential of the cones is faster (begins sooner and ends more quickly) than that of the rods (Brown et al, 1965). A pure cone (photopic) response is obtained if the retina is first sufficiently light adapted to saturate the rods. A pure rod (scotopic) response is obtained if the retina is well dark adapted and stimulated with light too dim to excite cones. Rods and cones may also be excited simultaneously (mesopic response). Thus the receptors generate a cornea-positive voltage, the waveform of which depends on whether it is driven by rods, cones, or both rods and cones.

The Müller cell is the major postreceptor cell that is a source of the ERG, although some contribution probably comes from bipolar cells, which also have a radial orientation of processes. These postreceptor sources generate a positive voltage at the cornea. The ERG thus results from the algebraic summation of an initial cornea, negative potential and a later cornea-positive potential. The leading edge of the negative potential (from the receptors) forms the a-wave of the ERG. The positive potential (postreceptor cells) forms the b-wave. Since these waves are of opposite polarity, delay in onset of the b-wave without change in its amplitude results in an apparent increase in the a-wave.

The mixing of rod and cone receptor potentials with rod and cone driven postreceptor potentials at the cornea results in a variety of ERG waveforms whose character depends on stimulus conditions. A practical recording procedure starts with a rapidly (3 Hz) repeated flash that is well above cone threshold and with the eye light adapted. This produces a standard photopic ERG. The patient is then dark adapted and the scotopic ERG is recorded with a slowly repeated dim flash (0.3 Hz) that is well below cone threshold. Finally, flash intensity is raised to above cone thresholds, but the eye remains relatively dark adapted as the stimulus frequency is still 0.3 Hz. This produces the mesopic response. Although some laboratories emphasize the rod and cone responses by using blue or red stimuli, it is not necessary in most patients. Colored stimuli are useful to separate cone from rod responses in patients with elevated rod thresholds.

The ERG is evaluated as to waveform and amplitude. The waveform measures that are most helpful are the implicit times of the a- and b-waves, that is, the time lapse from the stimulus to the peak of the a- or b-wave. A second waveform consideration is the relative prominence of a- and b-waves. Since these waves are the result of summation of voltages of opposite polarity, reduction of one causes an apparent enhancement of the other. The most common ERG abnormality is reduction of b-wave amplitude without reduction of the a-wave. This ERG waveform appears to have a larger than normal a-wave; it is "shifted to negativity." This shift may occur in all degrees from slight to total, in which case the ERG consists of an isolated receptor potential that is totally negative. The normal ERG a- and b-waves may be compared conveniently by calculating their ratio (Pearlman, 1981). Reduction of the b/a ratio occurs in all generalized retinal diseases that involve postreceptor processes (e.g., diabetic retinopathy) or transmission from receptor to postreceptor processes (e.g., retinitis pigmentosa or congenital stationary night blindness).

"White-Noise" (Random Flash) ERG

The ERG has been an important research tool of the visual physiologist and psychophysicist for nearly half a century. The usefulness of data obtained by the technique as presently used is limited by its inter- and intrasubject variability and by the crudeness of data interpretation. Thus, the utility of the ERG would be improved if it were practical to collect more data in a recording session of reasonable length and if it were possible to detect, in a reliable manner, subtle changes indicative of alteration of retinal function. What is needed is a recording method which permits continuous data collection and a technique of data analysis capable of resolving minimal functional changes with good reliability. These are the attributes of the "white-noise" analysis first applied to a biological preparation by Marmarelis and Naka (1972; 1973) and to the human ERG by Koblasz (1978).

Nonlinear analysis of limited usefulness has previously been applied to the ERG. Troelstra and Schweitzer (1968) produced a nonlinear ERG model with the use of paired flashes. The technique has been used clinically but generally is not suitable for patient use since the subject must not blink after the first flash. The stimuli also are nonphysiologic. The synchronous detector technique of Fricker and Sanders (1975) avoids some of the variability inherent in the usual ERG recording method, but it is time consuming if many stimulus frequencies are to be used and does not provide information about waveform. Fricker and Sanders also have used a rapid random-flash method, that is in some respects analogous to the white-noise technique in that cross-correlation of input and output is accomplished and used to derive amplitude and phase measurements of the response. The procedure can be done quickly, does not provide a canonical (single) response description, and uses a nonphysiologic stimulus -- limitations that are circumvented by the white-noise method (Fricker and Sanders, 1975).

The "white noise" input is a full-field light stimulus that varies "randomly" in intensity, seeming to flicker or twinkle. The mean intensity can be varied to obtain scotopic or photopic recordings. The interval of continuous random stimulation lasts 1 minute; repetition of the stimulus is unnecessary. An alternative, more powerful stimulus is the "binary flash." A flash is or is not presented every few milliseconds with a 50% probability. Larger potentials are evoked but the stimulus is less physiologic. The minimum interval between flashes is not critical, although the smaller the interval, the better the time resolution of the system. An interval of 16 ms works quite well.

The analysis consists of cross-correlating the output, at discrete intervals, with the input, at discrete intervals. The data are then reduced to a matrix of correlation values that represent the history of the influence of the preceding randomly varying input on the output. It is convenient to plot this table of values as a contour map. The mathematical formulation on which white-noise analysis is based is a series expansion in which the first term gives rise to the "first order kernel" and represents the linear properties of the system. The second and following (higher order) kernels represent its nonlinear properties. Thus, each term of the expansion may be used to derive a table of values or a contour map. This analysis, since it relates input to output in a canonical manner, lends itself to modeling of the system. The derived kernels can be used to reconstruct the response to a single flash of light. Such a plot of the first-order kernel approximately resembles the usual ERG. If a plot of the second-order kernel impulse response is added to the first, the approximation to the single-flash ERG is very close. Thus, it is only necessary to calculate first-and second-order kernels to characterize the ERG with considerable mathematical precision (Ogden et al, 1980) (Fig. 5.2).

This characterization contains a great deal of information that can be translated into amplitude, latencies, phase shifts, power density spectra, etc, for comparison with previously recorded data. This is the basis of the claim that it may permit detection of subtle differences in retinal function.

Of greater importance is the fact that with the use of Volterra kernels (which are derived from Wiener kernels) mean light levels have little effect on the results of the analysis as long as function is clearly within a specified range of intensities (i.e., scotopic, mesopic, or photopic). This property of the analysis will result in much less intersubject variation.

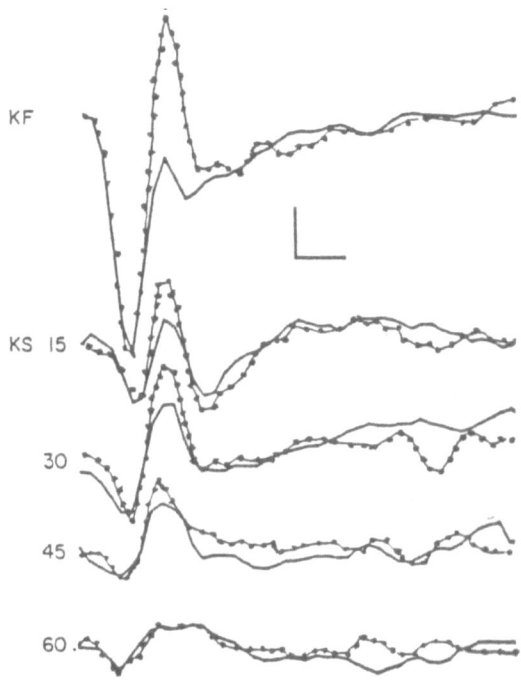

Figure 5.2. First - (KF) and second - order kernels (KS) recorded before (.....) and 126 days after surgery (____) from one animal. The cuts through the KS were made at 15-, 30-, 45-, and 60-ms flash intervals. Calibration: preoperative KF; 2.7 μV; postoperative KF; 1.1 μV; preoperative KS; 1.1 μV; postoperative KS; 0.44 μV. Time, 28 ms. (redrawn with permission of Ogden et al, 1980).

In practice, use of white-noise analysis is limited by the small size of the recorded potentials and by the limited ability of the retina to respond to high-frequency stimulation. Although providing excellent ERGs from relatively normal retina, the technique may be unusable in the severely diseased retina. For instance, many patients with retinitis pigmentosa and abnormal but recordable single flash ERGs have nonrecordable white-noise ERGs.

If the white-noise ERG is actually recordable, it may contain information not available in the single-flash ERG. For instance, the ratio of first-order to second-order kernel magnitude changes reversibly in the presence of vitreous hemorrhage. Also, the effect of vitreous blood and ocular trauma on the flash and white-noise ERGs differs substantially. Depression of the latter lasts much longer. The standard ERG recovers from the effect of vitreous blood in about 4 months in a primate trauma model at a time when the first-order kernel continues to show substantial abnormality (Mandelbaum et al, 1980).

The standard ERG may not be of use in assessing retinal function in cases of ocular trauma with a dense vitreal opacity. In this situation two tests have been

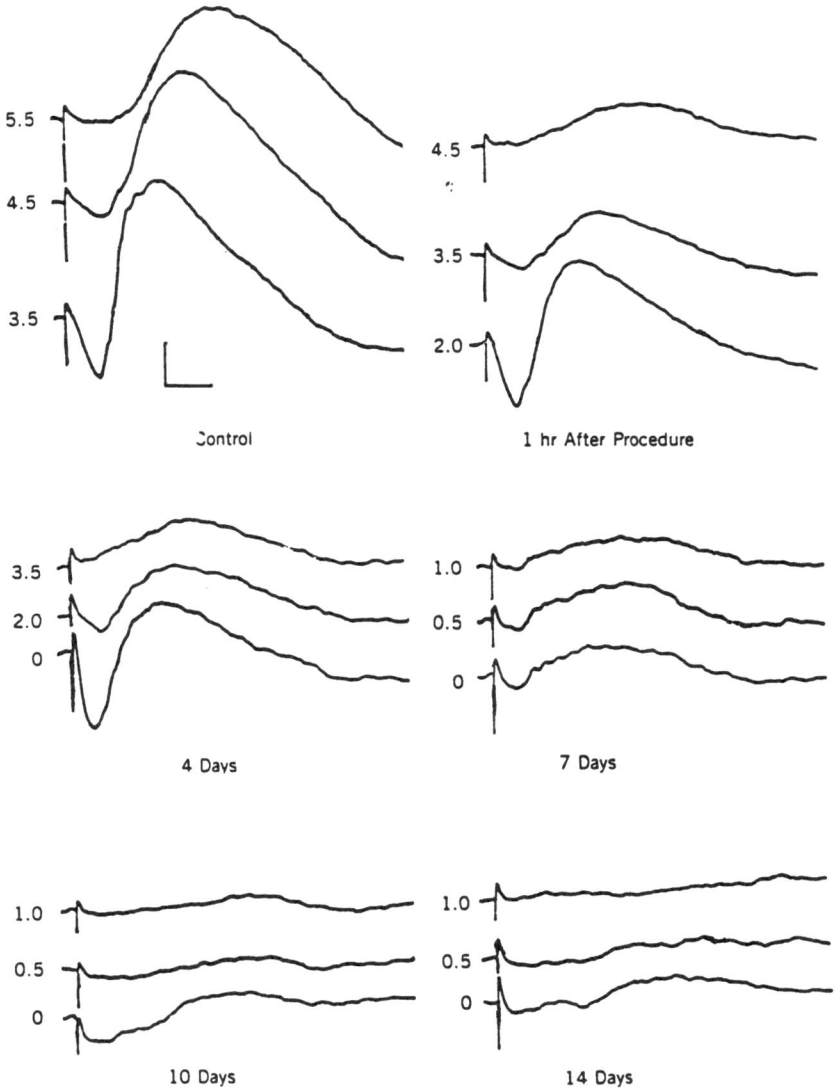

Figure 5.3. Electroretinogram recorded before and at various times following standard penetrating ocular injury and injection of 0.05 mL of autologous blood. Relative log attenuation of bright-flash stimulus is indicated for each trace. At 4 days, a-waves similar to the control could be evoked with 100 to 1,000 times more light, but b-wave was severely depressed. Calibration $50 \mu V$; 20 ms. (redrawn with permission from Mandelbaum et al, Arch Ophthalmol 98:1823-1828;1980 AMA).

developed to assess function behind the opacity: the bright-flash ERG and the electrically evoked ERG (EERG).

Bright-Flash ERG

The bright-flash ERG is a very useful test in selected patients. The test involves the use of a photographic strobe light with an intensity 10,000 to 100,000 times greater than the standard photopic stimulus. This test is appropriate for stimulation through the eyelids or for patients with almost opaque media. Its most frequent use is in patients with vitreous hemorrhage usually associated with trauma or diabetic retinopathy (Abrams and Knighton, 1982).

The object of the test is to obtain a saturated response, i.e., a response the amplitude of which does not increase with a 10-fold increase in light intensity. A series of responses are obtained using intensities that increase in 10-fold steps. The test is halted when the higher intensity fails to increase response amplitude. A normal response shows a striking decrease in a-wave latency with increased intensity and a sharply falling a-wave with a prompt return to the baseline, which is actually due to the b-wave. A slowed return to the baseline indicates b-wave reduction, a common finding in eyes containing blood and not a reliable indicator of retinal damage or detachment in these circumstances (Mandelbaum et al, 1980). If a saturated a-wave is obtained, useful information about the total area of functional retina is provided. Amplitude reduction with a normal crisp waveform suggests retinal detachment proportional to the reduction. Slowing of the waveform suggests retinal abnormality and atrophy if the amplitude is also reduced. Prospects for successful restoration of function by vitrectomy are poor in eyes with abnormal bright-flash ERGs, and the surgery is probably contraindicated in eyes with a nonrecordable bright flash ERG.

An important exception to this generalization is the eye with vitreous hemorrhage associated with a penetrating ocular injury. In such cases the vitreous may be replaced with blood, and this results in a media opacity of more than 6 log units optical density (Mandelbaum, 1980). Such eyes may fail to respond simply because the bright flash cannot penetrate the opacity. This situation virtually does not occur in a closed eye into which only a relatively small amount of blood can enter. It is not uncommon for the patient classed as "no light perception" to exclaim with delight when confronted with the bright flash, thus providing immediate subjective witness of retained function.

EERG

Electrical stimulation of the retina evokes a delayed monophasic wave with a negative polarity in an extracellular intraretinal recording. This was first described in the fish retina by Motokawa (1959). Ogden and Brown (1964) extended these studies to the cynomolgus monkey. In addition to the large delayed negative response, they observed a small "early negative wave" and a prominent positive wave. The late negative wave is of particular interest because it has the same intraretinal voltage distribution as the b-wave of the ERG and is assumed to be an equivalent response following electrical stimulation (Knighton, 1975a,b).

Electrically evoked phosphenes have been suggested as a useful test of retinal damage following ocular trauma. Meier-Koll (1972) determined the threshold and best frequency for evoking phosphenes in normal subjects and in patients with a number of retinal abnormalities. He was successful in identifying retinal abnormality in a high percentage of patients. Similar studies by Yonemura and Ishisaka (1955) revealed important differences between normal subjects and a rod monochromat. The test, however, has not been used much clinically, perhaps because it is subjective, requiring a verbal response from the patient.

Electrical excitation of an ERG is technically possible but difficult and is not likely to become a useful clinical test.   This is because a useful response requires suprathreshold stimulation that is uncomfortable to the patient.   Such a stimulus causes a large stimulus artifact that is difficult to control and contaminates the short latency response.

Potts and Inoue (1968; 1969; 1970) used electrical stimulation of the eye to evoke a cortical potential analogous to the visual evoked response (VER) and corresponding to the electrical phosphene.   The response was a complex waveform of greater magnitude than the flash VER.   Although this test is not used clinically, it has obvious potential for use in patients with severe ocular trauma.

Electroretinogram tests of specific cell function have been developed to evaluate for the blue cones, the inner retina, and ganglion cells.

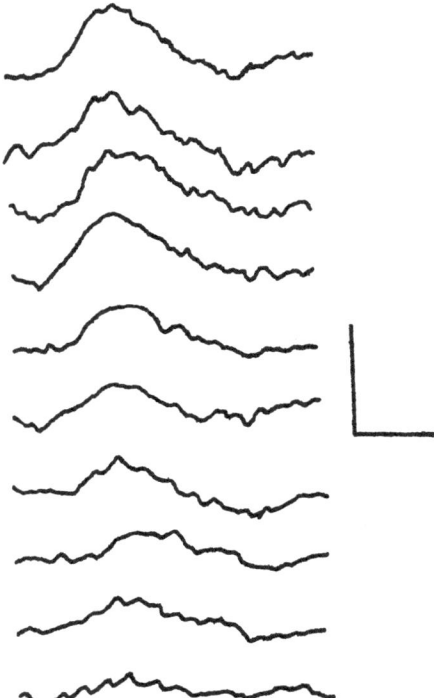

Figure 5.4. The ERG tracings for 10 normal obsevers to a 460/565 nm alternation at 1,600 troland. Calibration 30 μV; 50 ms (redrawn with permission from Sawusch et al, 1987).

Blue-Cone ERG

Blue-sensitive cones constitute only about 10% of retinal cones and generate much smaller and slower responses than the green- and red-sensitive cones.   Thus the blue-sensitive cones do not contribute significantly to the photopic ERG.   It is occasionally necessary to distinguish the rare blue-cone monochromat from the achromat so that an ERG test of blue-sensitive cones could be useful. Chromatic adaptation is not helpful because it reduces the sensitivity of the blue sensitive cones too severely.

Sawusch et al (1987) successfully isolated a blue-sensitive cone ERG by the use of "silent substitution": a stimulus that rapidly alternates in color between blue and yellow is adjusted to provide equal excitation and no ERG of the green cones. Such a stimulus is not at all balanced for the blue-sensitive cones that generate a blue-cone ERG (Fig 5.4). The waveform resembles a rod b-wave, but was shown to be generated by the blue-sensitive cones by spectral sensitivity studies. Adaptation was sufficient to saturate the rods but not the blue-sensitive cones.

Fluorescein ERG

Because the inner retinal layers are susceptible to ischemia, two electrophysiology tests may be useful in evaluating its function: the fluorescein ERG and oscillatory potentials.

Tamai and Mizuno (1981) noticed that the ERG of patients with background diabetic retinopathy was increased for up to 10 minutes after fluorescein intravenous injection. This effect was not seen in normal subjects. Their suggestion that secondary emission from leaked fluorescein increased the effective photon output from a flash seems reasonable. This test would seem to be a sensitive indicator of increased permeability to fluorescein. We have confirmed that the effect is absent in normal subjects and present in diabetics with retinopathy as stated by the authors, but we have not used the test further.

Oscillatory Potentials

Oscillatory potentials were first described by Cobb and Morton (1954). They are often described as "wavelets superimposed on the b-wave of the conventional ERG." Optimal recording of these wavelets can be found using a bright, slowly flickering flash with high-pass filtering (100-160 Hz).

The oscillatory potentials are depressed in conditions that cause widespread retinal ischemia, most notably diabetic retinopathy. Reduction of oscillatory potential amplitude may be used as a predictor of incipient deterioration of a retina with background diabetic retinopathy (Bresnick et al, 1984; Bresnick and Palta, 1987). At the present time, however, it is not the general practice to obtain repeated ERGs from diabetic patients.

The oscillatory potentials may also be abnormal in patients with glaucoma (Gur et al, 1987). This is perhaps not surprising since glaucoma is associated with degeneration of ganglion cells, and transsynaptic degeneration of inner nuclear layer cells is known to follow ganglion cell degeneration (Gills and Wadsworth, 1967). The oscillatory potentials are generated in the inner plexiform layer probably, at least in part, by amacrine cells (Yonemura and Kawasaki, 1981).

It has also been reported that oscillatory potentials are reduced in patients with X-L congenital stationary night blindness and in female carriers of X-linked recessive night blindness of this type (Miyake and Kawase, 1984; Heckenlively et al, 1983).

Pattern ERG

Evaluation of ganglion cells, the final output cells of the retina, has been elusive to electrophysiologists because ganglion cells do not contribute to the standard ERG. However, recent evidence has suggested that the pattern ERG may be a measure of ganglion cell function.

The first use of a pattern stimulus to evoke an ERG can probably be ascribed to Riggs et al (1964). One of the first clinical uses of patterned stimuli was probably that of

Lawwill (1974) who used an alternating bar pattern stimulus to selectively activate the macula. The advantage of this stimulus was that light scatter during phase alternation was constant; the only area actually stimulated was that on which the stimulus was imaged. The technique generated little interest, however, probably because its usefulness was limited to the macular ERG, and pattern stimulators were not generally available. There was little demand for focal ERG testing, and there was no suggestion that the pattern ERG differed fundamentally from the flash ERG.

It was not until evidence was presented that the pattern ERG represented the activity of ganglion cells that interest in this test became widespread. By 1981, use of alternating patterns (checkerboards) to evoke the VER was commonplace, and pattern stimulators were found in most clinical laboratories. The report of Maffei and Fiorentini (1981) that an ERG could be evoked by an alternating checkerboard pattern and that the response disappeared gradually following section of the optic nerve generated a great deal of interest. For the first time, an objective technique to evaluate the function of ganglion cells seemed at hand. The response was shown to be retina-dependent, since it was abolished by retinal ischemia (Maffei and Fiorentini, 1982). The loss of the response in the cat (Hollander et al, 1984) and monkey (Maffei et al, 1985) paralleled the gradual loss of ganglion cells killed by sectioning the optic nerve.

These initial reports led to widespread investigation of the pattern ERG as a method for evaluating ganglion cell degeneration, despite several cautionary papers showing that the response was at least partly attributable to the luminance or flash ERG.

When an alternating checkerboard pattern is used as a stimulus, the response represents the summation of "on" responses from the illuminated squares and "off" responses from the darkened squares. Each illuminated square generates a local ERG complete with a- and b-waves; each darkened square generates off-responses of opposite polarity. These responses are large and can be easily evaluated in isolation by appropriate stimulus paradigms. If the on- and off-responses are exactly equal in amplitude and opposite in polarity, they will sum to zero at the cornea. Any asymmetry in on- and off-responses will result in a recordable corneal ERG, but it will be a luminance ERG, independent of the pattern contrast per se, not generated by ganglion cells, and insensitive to ganglion cell disease.

Several studies have found that the pattern ERG amplitude is spatially tuned, i.e., a midrange of check sizes produces the greatest amplitude; larger or smaller check sizes produce smaller responses. This property is dependent on the field size, mean luminance, and retinal eccentricity of the pattern (Fiorentini et al, 1981; Odom et al, 1982; Korth, 1983; Korth and Rix, 1985). This evidence is considered to support the claim that the pattern ERG differs fundamentally from the flash ERG. Not all authors agree that the pattern ERG is spatially tuned (Armington et al, 1971; Kirkham and Coupland, 1983). The strongest evidence that the pattern ERG is different from the luminance ERG is its reduction following ganglion cell degeneration. Several studies cast doubt on the claim that the pattern ERG is generated solely by ganglion cells (Spekreijse, 1973; Blondeau et al, 1987; Riemslag et al, 1985; Harrison et al, 1987; Ringo et al, 1984; Sherman, 1982) and is totally contrast as opposed to luminance dependent (Ohzawa and Freeman, 1985).

Perhaps the most careful experimental study of the pattern ERG is that of Sieving and Steinberg (1985) who recorded the response with microelectrodes in the cat retina. They found the response to be maximal in amplitude in the inner retina (Arden et al 1982) and suggest, that the asymmetries between the responses of on- and off-stimulated retinal areas that sum to produce the corneal pattern response represent a contribution from Müller cells (Sieving and Steinberg, 1985) and the proximal negative response (PNR) described in the monkey by Ogden (1973).

The PNR is a highly local intraretinal response. It is detected by extracellular microelectrodes and is evoked by a small spot of light. The PNR is a sharply phasic wave of short duration at the onset and offset of illumination. The on- and off-PNR are not equal in size. It was suggested by Fatechand (1971) that the PNR is represented in the flash ERG. The time course of the PNR does not resemble the pattern ERG. A second intraretinal potential, the M (for Müller)-wave, has a time course similar to the pattern ERG and was shown by Sieving and Steinberg (1985) to behave like the pattern response in simulations of the latter.

The pattern ERG evoked by sinusoidal alternation of a checkerboard shows doubling in frequency. This could indicate that the response is based on nonlinear elements of the predominantly linear luminance response (Baker and Hess, 1984).

Regardless of uncertainty about the generator or generators of the pattern ERG, a preponderance of reports show changes in the response in patients with glaucoma (Wanger and Persson, 1983; Bobak et al, 1983; Trick, 1986; Marx et al, 1986), optic neuritis (Bobak et al, 1983; Vaegan and Billson, 1987; Plant et al, 1986), optic atrophy (Maffei and Fiortini, 1981; Maffei et al, 1985; Celesia and Kaufman, 1985; Dawson et al, 1982; Fiorentini et al, 1981; Harrison et al, 1987; Hollander et al, 1984), maculopathy (Celesia and Kaufman, 1985; Sherman, 1982), amblyopia (Arden and Wooding, 1985), early diabetic retinopathy (Arden and Wooding, 1985), and as a result of aging (Celesia et al, 1987; Trick et al, 1986). These conditions, except perhaps for senescence, have in common the loss of ganglion cells.

At the present time, the pattern ERG is not used in most clinical ERG laboratories. Standards for its evaluation are not available, and there is disagreement concerning the affect of repetition rate, luminance, contrast, and check size. It is obviously of most value if there is a normal fellow eye for comparison. As experience with the test accrues and instrumentation improves, it is likely that this test will be of substantial value in the assessment of optic nerve function.

Several points can be made concerning recording of this response. It is usually recorded with gold-foil electrodes to maintain good optical clarity. These are subject to blink artifact so prolonged averaging may be necessary for adequate noise elimination. The signals are small, 1 to 2 μV, and -- as clearly shown by the low-signal-to-noise ratios of many published examples -- difficult to record.

Most commercial television pattern generators have an appreciable luminance shift with each frame and are not suitable for use as pattern ERG stimulators. It seems likely that some of the conflicting results in the literature are the result of contamination of the pattern stimulus with a luminance shift. This would cause the recorded potential to be primarily a luminance ERG, which is well known to be unaffected by optic atrophy and ganglion cell degeneration.

From a pragmatic point-of-view, it matters little whether ganglion cells actually generate the pattern ERG if it can be clearly shown that the response is depressed in optic atrophy. Transsynaptic degeneration involving cells of the inner nuclear layer is a well-described consequence of ganglion cell degeneration (Gills and Wadsworth, 1967). This degeneration could well cause subtle changes in the on- or off-waveforms of the ERG and a decrease in the pattern ERG. If the response depends even indirectly on the integrity of ganglion cells, it has potential as a clinical test.

Careful experimental studies are required to establish the nature of this response. But such studies should be done in mammals. Results of investigations in the pigeon (Bagnoli et al, 1984; Blondeau et al, 1987), for example, are not readily extrapolated to primates. The bird inner retina is avascular, dependent on the pecten for its supplies of oxygen.

Focal ERG and VEP

The standard ERG is a summed potential across the entire retina. Small areas of abnormal function will not significantly alter the ERG. For example, in patients with macular degeneration, the ERG appears to be normal, since the macula only constitutes a small area of the retina. Focal techniques have been developed to assess function in discrete retinal areas.

The standard flash-ERG response is the algebraic sum of potentials generated over the entire retina. The amplitude of the flash ERG is proportional to the area of stimulated retina (Brindley and Westheimer, 1965). The macular region, often of particular interest to the ophthalmologist, accounts for only about 1% of the retinal area. Thus, the flash ERG is typically normal in retinal diseases that involve only the macula.

Various techniques for the recording of activity from localized areas of the retina in research settings have been discussed. It has not been until recently that recording focal ERGs and VEPs has been feasible in a clinical setting because of the small retinal signal and difficulty in maintaining fixation.

The recording of focal ERGs was first discussed more than 50 years ago. Cooper et al (1933) attempted to compare the response of the macula with that of the periphery (30° from fixation). The macular response was slightly larger in amplitude but similar in waveform compared with the periphery. Other early attempts to record from selected areas (Crampton and Armington, 1955) also found no differences in response across the retina.

The need to control for stray light was demonstrated independently by Asher (1951) and Boynton and Riggs (1951). They found that stimuli centered on the optic nerve head produced a large amplitude ERG from light-scatter. The aforementioned studies (Cooper et al, 1933; Crampton and Armington, 1955) were confounded because they failed to control for these light scatter-effects. Thus, their recordings were not "focal" responses because light scatter would greatly enlarge the presumed area of retinal stimulation. In retrospect, they used stimulating conditions that maximized stray-light effects. Cooper et al (1933) tested subjects under completely dark-adapted conditions so that the peripheral retina would be more sensitive to stray light. Crampton and Armington (1955) used a large stimulus (19°).

Brindley and Westheimer (1965) reported a new technique for recording focal ERGs. They extended the ideas of Armington et al (1961) by using a hemispheric bowl with adapting lights of greater intensity. The stimulus could be varied in size and/or intensity and presented anywhere within the visual field on the bowl against a bright adapting surround. They used a number of controls to demonstrate that stray-light effects were negligible on their ERGs.

Arden and Bankes (1966) followed up this study in the clinical setting. They reported a case in which a patient with unilateral macular degeneration had a normal macular ERG in the good eye and a nonrecordable macular ERG in the affected side.

While these early studies demonstrated that focal responses could be measured in the research setting, their clinical applicability was unsatisfactory owing to the inability of most patients to fixate a target reliably. Ideally, direct visual control of the stimulus is desirable, since the patient may be noncooperative or unable to maintain fixation because of poor vision. A number of investigators modified ophthalmic equipment such as the pleoptophor (Shipley, 1969), the ophthalmoscope (Sandberg et al, 1977), the biomicroscope (Hirose et al, 1977), and the fundus camera (Miyake et al, 1981) to allow visualization of the stimulus while recording. The development of these systems (mainly the Sandberg et al, 1977, and Miyake et al, 1981, systems) has led to a number of papers dealing with the focal ERGs and/or VEPs in the clinical setting.

Sandberg et al (1977) used a modified direct ophthalmoscope to record macular VEPs in 47 patients with macular scars, macular degenerations, or retinitis pigmentosa. They found that all 31 patients with visual acuity 20/50 or less had abnormal VEPs. All 6 patients with macular degenerations and 5 of 10 with retinitis pigmentosa also showed abnormal focal VEPs. Sandberg et al (1979) found abnormal focal ERGs in all patients with juvenile macular degenerations and visual acuity worse than 20/50. In patients with retinitis pigmentosa , they found that 5 of 5 patients with visual acuity 20/40 or less and only 3 of 11 patients with visual acuity 20/30 or better had abnormal focal ERGs. Jacobson et al (1979) found normal macular ERGs in patients with strabismic amblyopia. Birch and Fish (1988) have used this instrument to show a decrease of macular response with age and in macular diseases.

Miyake and Awaya (1984), using a modified nonmydriatic fundus camera, also found normal focal ERGs in patients with amblyopia. Horiguchi et al (1986) reported flash and focal ERGs from a pair of siblings with Best's disease. They demonstrated normal flash ERGs and absent macular ERGs.

Other investigators have continued to use focal electrophysiology in basic and clinical research. One group has used a rear projection system or a television screen to record macular ERGs and VEPs (Arden and Vaegan, 1983; Vaegan et al, 1984; Vaegan and Billson, 1986). Another group has used an array of light-emitting diodes in a ganzfeld bowl for focal stimulation in explorations of the temporal modulation transfer function (Seiple et al, 1986a) and in patients with retinal degenerations (Seiple et al, 1986b). These techniques do not allow for visualization of the stimulus on the retina while recording, and are therefore not suitable for use in the usual clinical population, where few patients are capable of reliably precise fixation for extended periods of time.

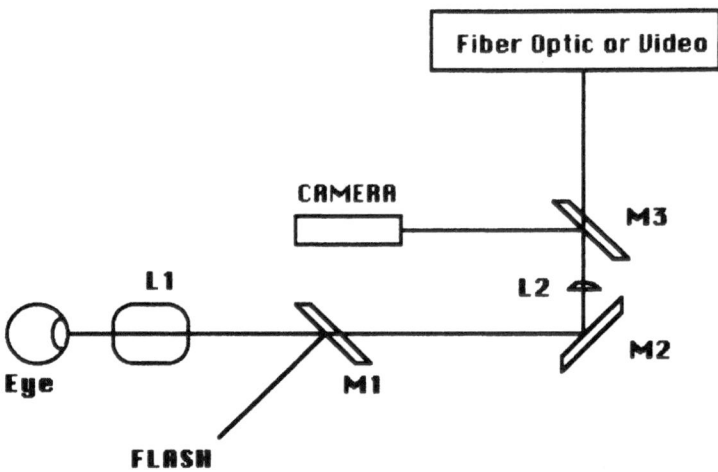

Figure 5.5. Schematic of optical system for focal stimuli. M1,3 half-silvered mirrors, M2 full-silvered mirror; L1-2, lens systems.

Current Study

We have developed and begun testing a system similar to that described by Miyake et al (1981). The system utilizes a nonmydriatic Canon fundus camera with a channel added to provide either a pattern stimulus or a flash stimulus on an annulus background. The system uses infrared light to provide a constant video monitor view of the fundus and permits direct visual control of placement of a small spot or pattern stimulus. (Fig 5.5)

Methods

Observation and Stimulation System

The stimulus source is a xenon flash controlled by an electronic stimulator (Grass SD-9). The stimulus is led to the fundus camera via a concentric 2-channel fiber optic placed in the plane of the internal fixation device. The surround is variable in intensity and controlled by a tungsten source with a blue-green filter. An auxiliary fixation target is attached to the side of the camera to be used for fixation by the fellow eye.

We have also used a checkerboard pattern as a stimulus. The checkerboard pattern is generated by an Apple IIe computer program (Hope et al, 1983) that allows manipulation of alternation rate and checkerboard size. This pattern is also delivered directly in the plane of the internal fixation light of the camera by a 1-inch video monitor. The angular subtense of the stimulus can be varied by placing masks over the monitor screen.

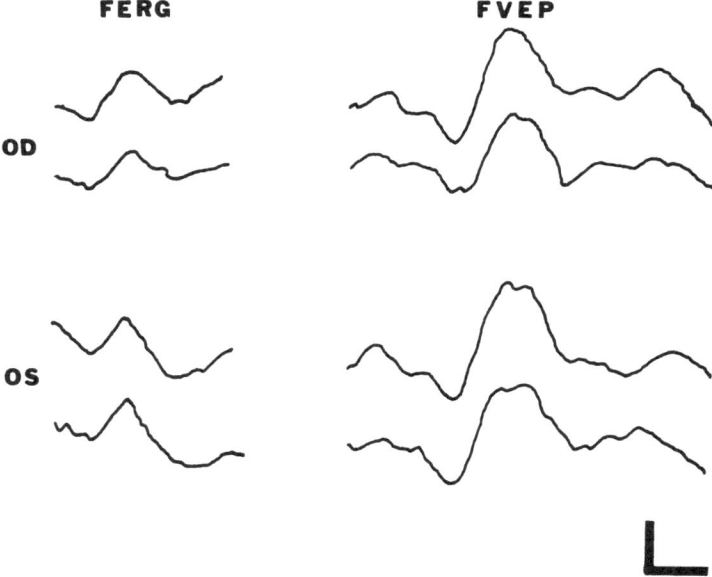

Figure 5.6. Repeated tracings of focal ERGs and VEPs from the right (OD) and left (OS) eyes. Note symmetry in responses. Calibration: $3 \mu V$, 50 ms.

Recording System of the ERG and VEP

Focal ERGs were recorded using either a clear Burian Allen electrode or a version of the gold-foil electrode. Although some authors have claimed that recording focal ERGs is hampered with the Burian Allen, we have had success with it. The VEP is recorded in the usual manner.

The signals are filtered (1-100 Hz) and averaged on a Nicolet Compac system. Usually 250 responses are averaged with a stimulus frequency of 3 Hz for the focal flash ERG/VEP and 3.5 reversals per second for the focal pattern VEP. An artifact rejection system eliminates transient signals larger than $100 \mu V$.

Results

A comparison of simultaneously measured focal ERGs and VEPs from a normal subject is shown in Figure 5.6. The stimulus was presented at 3 Hz with no background present. Note the symmetry in ERG and VEP responses. No response was recorded from the nerve head. We believe this lack of response is due to the superior imaging capabilities of the camera and controlled fixation of the stimulus on the nerve head. Continuing further along the visual pathway the VER will be discussed.

VER

The visual evoked response (VER), also called the visual evoked potential (VEP), is an electrical response of the visual cortex to an appropriate visual stimulus. The response is recorded with electrodes placed on the scalp in a manner similar to that of the electroencephalogram. For ophthalmic testing the electrodes are placed on the midline 1 cm above their inion and at the vertex. The inion electrode is approximately above the striate cortex and is in a position to sample both hemispheres equally. The vertex electrode is over cortex that is relatively silent to visual stimuli and is considered a reference. The VER is much smaller in amplitude than the spontaneous EEG activity. The evoked response is isolated from the random background activity by a process of computer averaging of repeated responses.

The Flash VER

The usual stimulus for the VER is a full-field flash delivered to one eye at a time. Thus the midline electrode detects activity from the nasal half of the stimulated retina conveyed to the contralateral cortex through the ipsilateral optic nerve and contralateral optic radiation. This activity is mixed with activity from the temporal half of the retina and conveyed to the ipsilateral cortex through the ipsilateral radiation. A normal response indicates that these structures are intact.

The flash VER has a complex waveform that varies substantially among different normal individuals. For this reason it is not an accurate measure of subtle changes in vision that involve both eyes. The VER is normally highly symmetric; stimulation of the left eye evokes a response that closely resembles the response evoked by stimulation of the right eye. Thus unilateral abnormality is much easier to detect with the flash VER than bilateral.

About 70% of the visual cortex in concerned with macular vision, so-called "cortical magnification." Thus macular abnormality has more impact on the VER than peripheral retinal abnormality. Unfortunately, the variability of the VER is sufficiently great that it may mask changes due to a macular lesion. For this reason the VER has been a disappointment as a preoperative predictor of macular function in patients with, for instance, dense cataracts. The VER is an excellent screening test of visual function in small infants and in patients with dense cataracts or vitreous hemorrhage. It is often abnormal in the presence of optic neuritis or other lesions along the visual pathway.

The Pattern Shift VER

A VER can also be evoked by a pattern stimulus, usually a black and white checkerboard pattern in which the black and white checks alternate about three times per second. The waveform of the pattern VER is much simpler and less variable among individuals than that produced by a flash. The typical response features a positive wave that peaks about 100 ms after the pattern shift and is called the P100 wave. The pattern shift VER is delayed in a high percentage of patients with optic neuritis. The delay often persists after the lesion has become asymptomatic. The response can be delayed in the presence of a visual pathway lesion of any type and does not distinguish between compressive lesions and optic neuritis.

The pattern VER is dependent on resolution of the visual stimulus. It provides an estimate of visual acuity if patterns of different visual subtense are used. The presence of a normal response to a small check size proves that the pattern was resolved and that the retina and central visual pathways concerned with its resolution are intact. It does not prove that the patient is sighted, since extensive bilateral pathology of the visual association areas can produce functional blindness in the presence of a normal response. The probability that such pathology exists without clinical indication is low; thus the pattern VER provides a reliable objective indicator of the general performance level of the optic nerve of which the cooperative patient should be capable.

VEPs to Laser-Generated Patterns

Laser interference fringes in combination with subjective assessment of contrast-sensitivity testing have been used to evaluate visual function (Cambell and Green, 1965). Laser interference fringes have the advantage of forming a retinal image independent of visual refraction. Thus, once the image is placed at the pupil plane, it will be in focus on the retina. The use of laser interference patterns has also been used in the subjective assessment of vision behind ocular opacities (Goldmann, 1972; Enoch et al, 1979; Goldmann et al, 1980). However, there must be a "window" through the opacity to project the fringes onto the retina (Goldmann et al, 1980). When opacities are present, fine fringes are masked by speckle patterns produced by light-scatter from the opacity.

Laser fringes have also been used to generate retinal (Krüger et al, 1982) and cortical (Arden and Sheorey, 1977; Sugimachi, 1979) potentials in normal and cataract patients. These potentials were found to be predictive in estimating postsurgery vision in some cases. However, as previously stated, laser fringe patterns require a transparent window around the opacity or laser speckle will result. This speckle pattern will cause an underestimate of visual acuity because it masks higher spatial frequencies more. However, a novel technique overcomes the problem with laser speckle; in fact, it measures the VEP produced by the speckle (Fukuhara et al, 1983). These investigators were able to reasonably predict visual function in unilateral cataracts by comparing the amplitudes of the laser speckle VEP between eyes and multiplying that ratio by visual acuity in the good eye.

Bright-Flash VER

Following a penetrating ocular injury with vitreous hemorrhage, the standard flash VER may be absent, suggesting total retinal detachment or loss of optic nerve function. This can be misleading if the hemorrhage is dense. The test should be repeated with the bright flash, a photographic strobe 10,000 to 100,000 times brighter than the standard flash. The bright flash is sufficiently intense to penetrate the high optical density of the vitreous blood and may produce a good response if the system is intact. In such cases the patient: often exclaims with delight that the stimulus is actually seen.

These standard techniques for measuring the VEP require extensive signal averaging and are thus difficult to perform in young children or inattentive adults. Two special techniques have been devised to assess posterior pathway function in such patients; use of sedation or hypnosis and sweep techniques.

Chloral Hydrate Sedation and the Pattern VER

The pattern VER is a very useful objective test of visual function in infants. Unfortunately, many infants are not testable under the usual laboratory conditions owing to their failure to regard the pattern stimulus. Wright et al (1986) have been able to record excellent pattern VERs from sleeping infants sedated with chloral hydrate (100 mg/kg). The infant is held facing the checkerboard stimulus and the lid of the tested eye gently elevated by the examiner. Providing a Bell's phenomenon is not present, reliable responses can be obtained to a variety of check sizes. As in all pattern testing, a normal response indicates in a general way the absence of gross pathology in the macula and its central projections. An abnormal response must be interpreted cautiously, particularly if bilateral and if in the presence of a normal flash response. This procedure, however, holds great promise for evaluation of amblyopia in infants and small children.

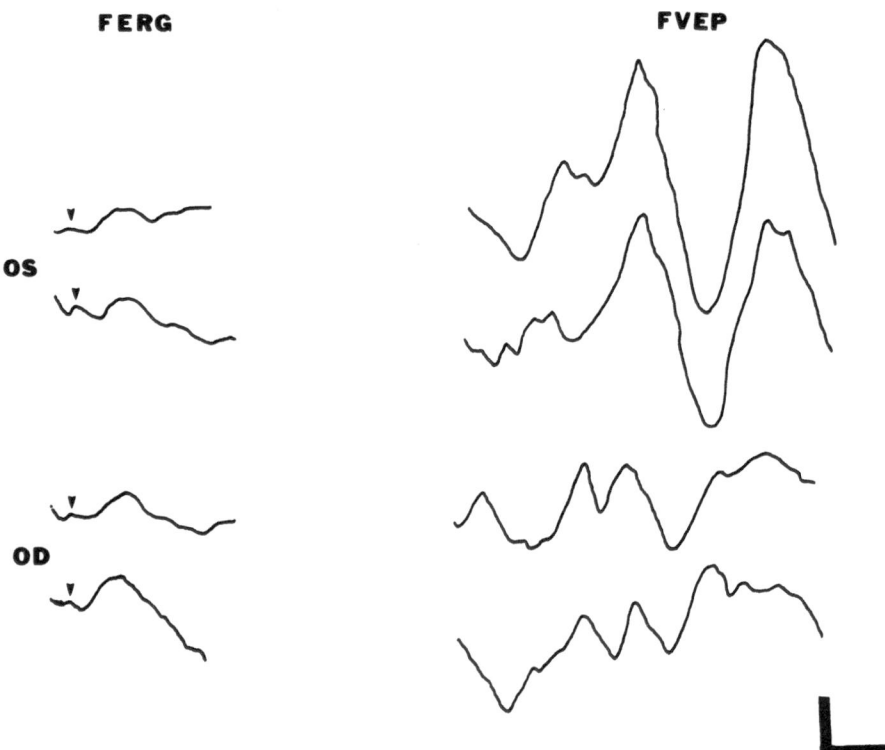

Figure 5.7. Right (OD) and left (OS) eye recordings of focal ERGs and VEPs. Note symmetry in focal ERG response and assymmetry in focal VEP response. This patient had 20/70 vision OS and 20/200 vision OD. Calibration 3 μV, 50 ms.

Sedation by Hypnosis

Chloral hydrate sedation works very well with small children and it is only rarely necessary to administer a general anesthesia to obtain ERG or VER recordings from such patients. Children weighing more than 60 pounds present rather more of a problem. Many older children with behavior problems who require sedation respond poorly, if at all, to safe doses of chloral hydrate.

Bogoslovsky et al (1973) describe the successful use of hypnosis in children older than 10 undergoing electroretinography with a contact lens electrode and topical anesthesia. Recordings were stable and the hypnosis stopped nystagnoid eye movements that otherwise would have interfered with the recordings. The limitation of the procedure is that hypnosis is difficult or impossible to induce in small children and in those with low suggestibility.

Sweep VEPs

The classic techniques of recording flash and pattern VEPs can require lengthy averaging to register a single response. If one uses a variety of stimulus conditions (e.g., in estimating visual acuity), the process is proportionately longer. The lengthy recording times are often not clinically practical for assessing function in children or for screening procedures.

A relatively recent development using "swept" stimuli has shown promise for rapid assessment of vision (Tyler et al, 1979; Seiple et al, 1984). The sweep technique uses a counterphasing sinusoidal or square-wave grating modulated at high temporal frequency while simultaneously changing (either high-to-low or low-to-high) the spatial frequency at a slow rate. The VEPs are recorded with narrow-band synchronous filter techniques. Using these procedures, acuity and contrast sensitivity have been assessed in young children.

Finally, some techniques developed for evaluating retinal function can also be used in assessing posterior pathway function. The electrically evoked VEP can be measured simultaneously with the EERG. Also, the focal VEP can be measured simultaneously with the focal ERG.

Figure 5.7 are eye tracings of a patient with visual acuities of 20/70 in the left eye and 20/200 in the right, with no significant fundus findings. The patient had normal full-field flash ERGs for each eye. Focal ERGs from the macula were also normal. Focal VEPs were asymmetric with a loss of amplitude in the right eye consistent with the patient's stated visual acuity.

Future of the Tests

Some of the test described as "new" have already been established as part of the standard protocol in some laboratories, e.g., oscillatory potentials and pattern ERGs. Other techniques appear to be better suited for research enviornments at present (DC-ERG, white-noise ERG, fluorescein ERG). Many of the other new tests may be applied in a number of research/clinical settings including:

1. Special visual analysis: If there is, for example, a question of RPE function, the stress tests may be more useful than the EOG. The blue-cone ERG may be applicable in objective assessment of blue-cone function. There is some evidence that suggests that some diseases may involve the blue-cone system, e.g., glaucoma (Adams et al, 1987). Focal ERGs and VEPs appear to be valuable in assessing macular function.

2. Assessment of visual function behind cloudy media: Bright-flash ERG/VEP; electrically evoked ERG/VEP, laser fringe/speckle ERG/VEP are all tests that have been used in prediction of visual function behind opacities.

3. Assessing vision in uncooperative patients: Eye-blink ERG requires little cooperation other than allowing normal light adaptation to occur. The focal ERG/VEP utilizes direct stimulus imaging; recording can thus be stopped when the subject loses fixation or tries to alter accommodation. Laser fringe/speckle stimulus by definition will be in focus on the retina if centered on the pupil.

4. Assessment of vision in children: Eye-blink EOG may have use because it requires little cooperation; in addition, the VEPs measured under sedation and sweep VEPs were designed for use in infants.

Summary

This chapter has presented a brief review of some of the new techniques for assessing the site of pathologic involvement of the sensory visual system. Table 5.1 is a review of old and new techniques for localizing disease along the visual pathways. This review only begins to explore some of the new techniques of electrodiagnostics. The authors apologize for techniques that may have been omitted. The field of clinical electrophysiology is constantly expanding and is sure to offer a number of new methods to provide an earlier, more accurate diagnosis of pathology as well as aid in monitoring treatment efficacy.

Table 5.1. Summary of old and new techniques for
localizing lesions along the sensory visual pathways

Area	Old	New
RPE	EOG	DC-ERG, eye-blink EOG, stress tests
Retina	ERG	White-noise ERG, bright-flash ERG, EERG
Blue cone	None	Blue-cone ERG
Inner retina	ERG	Oscillatory potentials, fluorescein ERG
Ganglion cells	VEP	Pattern ERG
Macula	VEP	Focal ERG/VEP
Higher visual pathways	VEP	Sedation, sweep VEP, Bright-flash electrically evoked VEP, focal VEP

References

Abrams GW, Knighton RW. Falsely extinguished bright-flash electroretinogram. Arch Ophthalmol 1982;100:1427-9.

Adams AS, Henon G, Husted R. Clinical measure of central visual function in glaucoma and ocular hypertension. Arch Ophthalmol 1987;105:782-7.

Arden GB, Bankes JLK. Foveal electroretinogram as a clinical test. Bri J Ophthalmol 1966; 50:740.

Arden GB, Barrada A. An analysis of the electro-oculograms of a series of normal subjects. Bri J Ophthalmol 1962;46:468-82.

Arden GB, Sheorey UB. The assessment of visual function in patients with opacities: a new evoked potential method using a laser interferometer. In Desmedt JE. (ed) Visual Evoked Potentials in Man: New Developments. Oxford: Clarendon Press:1977;pp. 381-94.

Arden GB, Vaegan. Electroretinograms evoked in man by local uniform or patterned stimulation. J Physiol 1983; 341:85-104.

Arden GB, Wooding SL. Pattern ERG in amblyopia. Invest Ophthalmol Vis Sci 1985; 26: 88-96.

Arden GB, Vaegan, Hogg CR. Clinical and experimental evidence tha the pattern electroretinogram (PERG) is generated in more proximal layers than the focal electroretinogram (FERG). Ann NY Acad Sci 1982; 388:580-601.

Armington JC, Corwin TR, Marsetta R. Simultaneously recorded retinal and cortical responses to pattern stimuli. J Opt Soc Am 1971; 61:1514-21.

Asher H. The electroretinogram of the blind spot. J Physiol 1951; 112:40P.

Bagnoli P, Porciatti V, Francesconi W, Barsellotti R. Pigeon pattern electroretinogram: a response unaffected by chronic section of the optic nerve. Exp Brain Res 1984; 55: 2253-262.

Baker CL Jr, Hess RF. Linear and nonlinear components of the human electroretinogram. J Neurophysiol 1984; 51: 952-67.

Birch DG, Fish GE. Focal cone electroretinogram: Aging and macular disease. Doc Ophthalmol 1988;69:211-20.

Blondeau P, Lamarche J, Lafond G, Brunette JR. Pattern electroretinogram and optic nerve section in pigeons. Curr Eye Res 1987; 6: 747-56.

Bobak P, Bodis-Wollner I, Harnois C, Maffei L, Mylin L, Podos S, Thorton J. Pattern elctroretinograms and visual evoked potentials in glaucoma and multiple sclerosis. Am J Ophthalmol 1983; 96:72-83.

Bogoglovsky AI, Kovalchuk NA, Makarenko YA. Method for electroretinographic investigations in children in a state of hypnotic sleep. Vis Res 1973; 13: 1767-9.

Boyton RM, Riggs LA. The effect of stimulus area and intensity on the human retinal response. J Exp Psychol 1951; 42: 217-26.

Bresnick GH, Palta M. Oscillatory potential amplitudes: relation to severity of diabetic retinopathy. Arch Ophthalmol 1987;105:929-33.

Bresnick GH, Korth K, Groo A, Palta M. Electroretinographic oscillatory potentials predict progression of diabetic retinopathy. Arch Ophthalmol 1984; 102: 1307-11.

Brindley GS, Westheimer G. The spatial properties of the human electroretinogram. J Physiol 1965; 179:518-36.

Brown KT. The electroretinogram: its components and their origins. Vis Res 1968; 8: 633-77.

Brown KT, Watanabe K. Isolation and identification of a receptor potential from the pure cone fovea of the monkey retina. Nature 1962a; 193: 958-60.

Brown KT, Watanabe K. Rod receptor potential from the retina of the night monkey. Nature 1962b; 196:547-50.

Brown KT, Watanabe K, Murakami M. The early and late receptor potentials of monkey cones and rods. Cold Spring Harbor Symp Quant Biol 1965; 30: 457-82.

Campbell F, Green DG. Optical and retinal factors affecting visual resolution. J Physiol 1965;181:576-93.

Carr RE, Siegel FM. Visual Electrodiagnostic Testing. Baltimore:Williams and Wilkins:1982.

Celesia GG, Kaufman D. Pattern ERGs and visual evoked potentials in maculopathies and optic nerve diseases. Invest Ophthalmol Vis Sci 1985; 26:726-35.

Celesia GG, Kaufman D, Cone S. Effects of age and sex on pattern electroretinograms and visual evoked potentials. Electroencephalogr Clin Neurophysiol 1987; 68: 161-71.

Cobb WA, Morton HB. A new component of the human electroretinogram. J Physiol 1954; 123: 36-7.

Cooper S, Creed RS, Granit R. A Note on the Retinal action potential of the human eye. J Physiol 1933; 79:185-93.

Crampton GH, Armington JC. Area-intensity relation and retinal location in he human electroretinogram. Ann Physiol. 1955; 181:47-53.

Dawson WW, Maida TM, Rubin ML. Human pattern-evoked retinal responses are altered by optic atrophy. Invest Ophthalmol Vis Sci 1982; 22: 796-803.

Denny D, Denny C. The eye blink electro-oculogram Bri J Ophthalmol 1984; 68: 225-8.

Dodt E. Beitrage zur elektrophysiologie des auges. I. Metteilung. Uber die sekundare erhebung im aktionspotential des menschlichen auges bei belichtung. Albrecht Von Graefes Arch Klin Exp Ophthalmol 1951; 151: 672-92.

DuBois Reymond E. Untersuchungen uber thierische electricitat. 1849; Berlin, vol2-1,256.

Enoch JM, Bedell HE, Kaufman HE. Interferometric visual acuity testing in anterior segment disease. Arch Ophthalmol 1979;97:1916.

Fatechand G. The two components of the vitreal-wave and its intravitreal localization. Vis Res 1971; 11: 489-500.

Fiorentini A, Maffei L, Pirchio M, Spinelli D, Porciatti V. The ERG in response to alternating gratings in patients with diseases of the peripheral visual pathway. Invest Ophthalmol Vis Sci 1981; 21:490-3.

Fricker SJ, Sanders JJ. A new method of cone electroretinography: the rapid random flash response. Invest Ophthalmol Vis Sci 1975; 14: 131-7.

Fukuhara J, Vozato H, Nojima S, Salishin M, Nakao S. Visual-evoked potential elicited by laser speckle patterns. Invest Ophthalmol Vis Sci 1983:24:1400-7.

Gills JP, Wadsworth JAC. Retrograde transsynaptic degeneration of the inner nuclear layer of the retina. Invest Ophthalmol Vis Sci 1967; 6: 437-48.

Goldmann H. Examination of the fundus of the cataractous eye. Am J Ophthalmol 1972;73:309.

Goldmann H, Chrenková A, Cornaro S. Retinal visual acuity in cataractous eyes. Determination with interference fringes. Arch Ophthalmol 1980;98:1778.

Gur M, Zeevi YY, Brelick M, Neuman E. Changes in the oscillatory potientials of the elctroretinogram in glaucoma. Curr Eye Res 1987; 6: 457-66.

Hanitzsch R, Hommer K, Bornschein H. Der nachweis langsamer potentiale im menschlichen ERG. Vis Res 1966; 6: 245-50.

Harrison JM, O'Connor PS, Young RSL, Kincaid M, Bentley R. The pattern ERG in man following surgical resection of the optic nerve. Invest Ophthalmol Vis Sci 1987; 28: 492-9.

Heckenlively JR, Martin DA, Rosenbaum AL. Loss of electroretinographic oscillatory potentials, optic atrophy, and dysplasia in congenital stationary night blindness. Am J Ophthalmol 1983;96:526-34.

Heilig P, Thaler A, Bornschein H. Pearlman JT (ed) Slow potential of ERG in hemeralopia congenita. 1973;Proc Xth ISCERG Symposium, pp. 219-24.

Hirose T, Miyake Y, Hara A. Simultaneous recording of electroretinogram and visual evoked response. Arch Ophthalmol 1977; 95:1205-8.

Hollander H, Bisti S, Maffei L, Hebel R. Electroretinographic responses and retrograde changes of retinal morphology after intracranial optic nerve section. Exp Brain Res 1984; 55: 483-93.

Hope GW, Dawson WW, Odom JV. Microcomputer presentation of patterned stimuli for visual electrophysiology. In Kolder EJW (ed) Slow Potentials and Microprocessor Applications. Boston: Dr W Junk Publisher:1983.

Horiguchi M, Miyake Y, Yagasaki K. Local macular ERG in patients with Best's disease. Doc Ophthalmolo 1986; 63:325-31.

Jacobson SG, Sandberg MA, Effron MH, Berson EL. Foveal cone electroretinograms in strabismic amblyopia. Trans Ophthalmol Soc UK 1979; 99:353-6.

Kirkham TH, Coupland SG. The pattern ERG in optic nerve demyelination. Can J Neurol Sci 1983; 10: 256-60.

Knave B, Nilsson SEG, Lunt T. The human electroretinogram: d.c. recordings at low, conventional stimulus intensities. Description of a new method for clinical use. Acta Ophthalmol 1973; 51: 716-26.

Knighton RW. An electrically evoked slow; potential of the frog's retina. I. Properties of response. J Neurophysiol 1975a;38:185-209.

Knighton RW. Modification of the frog's electroretinogram by transretinal direct Current. J Neurophysiol 1975b;38:210-16.

Koblasz AJ. Nonlinearities of the human ERG reflected by Wiener kernels. Biol Cybern 1978; 31: 187-91.

Korth M. Pattern evoked, luminance evoked responses in the human electroretinogram. J Physiol 1983; 337:451-69.

Korth M, Rix R Changes in spatial selectivity of pattern ERG components with stimulus contrast. Albrecht Von Graefes Arch Klin Exp Ophthalmol 1985; 223:23-8.

Krüger CJ, Kusel R, Baier M, Rassow B. Retinal potentials evoked by alternating laser interference fringes. Doc Ophthalmol Proc Ser 1982;31:43-50.

Kühne W, Steiner J. Uber electrische vorgange im sehorgane. Unters Physiol Inst Univ Heidelberg 1881; 4: 64-160.

Lawwill T. The bar-pattern electroreinogram for clinical evaluation of the central retina. Am J Ophthalmol 1974; 78: 121-6.

Linsenmeier RA, Steinberg RH. Mechanisms of Azide induced increases in the c-wave and standing potential of the intact cat eye. Vis Res 1987;27:1-8.

Maffei L, Fiorentini A. Electroretinographic responses to alternating gratings before and after section of the optic nerve. Science 1981; 211: 953-5.

Maffei L, Fiorentini A. Electroretinographic responses to alternating gratings in the cat. Exp Brain Res 1982; 48: 327-34.

Maffei L, Fiorentini A, Bisti S, Hollander H. Pattern ERG in the monkey after section of the optic nerve. Exp Brain Res 1985; 59: 423-5.

Mandelbaum S, Cleary PE, Ryan SJ, Ogden TE. Bright-flash electroretinography and vitreous hemorrhage. Arch Ophthalmol 1980; 98:1823-1828.

Marmarelis PZ, Naka K-I. Non linear analysis of receptive-field responses in the catfish retina. I. Horizontal cell to ganglion cell chain. J Neurophys 1973; 36: 605-18.

Marmarelis PZ, Naka K-I. White noise analysis of a neuron chain: an application of Weiner theory. Science 1972; 175:1276-8.

Marx MS, Podos SM, Bodis-Wollner I, et al. Flash and pattern electroretinograms in normal and laser-induced glaucomatous primate eyes. Invest Ophthalmol Vis Sci 1986; 27: 378-86.

Matsuo F, Peters JF, Reilly EL. Electrical phenomena associated with movements of the eyelid. Electroencephalog Klin Neurophysiol 1975; 38: 507-11.

Meier-Koll A. Differentialdiagnose von Retinaschaden mittels elecktrisch evozierter Lichtempfindungen. Albrecht Von Graefes Arch Klin Exp Ophthalmol 1972;184:177-92.

Miller SS, Steinberg RH. Active transport of ions across frog retinal pigment epithelium. Exp Eye Res 1977a; 25: 235-48.

Miller SS, Steinberg RH. Passive ionic properties of frog retinal pigment epithelium. J Membr Biol 1977b; 36: 337-72.

Miyake Y, Awaya S. Stimulus deprivation amblyopia. Arch Ophthalmol 1984; 102:998-1003.

Miyake Y, Kawase Y. Reduced amplitude of oscillatory potentials in female carriers of X-linked recessive congenital stationary night blindness. Am J Ophthalmol 1984;98:208-15.

Miyake Y, Yanagida K, Kondo T, Yagasaki K, Ohta I. Subjective scotometry and recording of local electroretinogram and visual evoked response-system with television monitor of the fundus. Jpn J Ophthalmol 1981; 25:438-48, .

Motokawa M. Responses of retinal network to electrical stimulation. Tohoku J Exp Med 1959; 71: 41-53.

Niemeyer G. Light modulation of the standing potential in the perfused mammalian eye: characteristics and responses to acidosis. Doc Ophthalmol Proc Ser 1983;37:41-9.

Nilsson SEG, Skoog K. Covariation of the simultaneously recorded c-wave and standing potential of the human eye. Acta Ophthalmol 1975;53:721-30.

Noell WK. Studies on the electrophysiology and metabolism of the retina. 1953; Air university school of aviation medicine. Project report No 1.

Odom VJ, Maida TM, Dawson WW. Pattern-evoked retinal responses (PERR) in human: Effects of spatial frequency, luminance, and defocus. Curr Eye Res 1982; 2:99-108.

Ogden TE. The proximal negative response of the primate retina. Vis Res 1973; 13:797-807.

Ogden TE, Brown KT. Intraretinal responses of the cynamologous monkey to electrical stimulation of the optic nerve and retina. J Neurophysiol 1964; 27: 682-705.

Ogden TE, Larkin RM, Fender DF, Cleary PE, Ryan SJ. The use of non-linear analysis of the primate ERG to detect retinal dysfunction. Exp Eye Res 1980; 31: 381-8.

Ohzawa I, Freeman RD. Pattern evoked potentials from the cat's retina. J Neurophysiol 1985; 54: 691-700.

Perlman I. Relationship between the amplitudes of the b wave and the a wave as a useful index for evaluating the electroretinogram. Bri J Ophthalmol 1981; 67: 443-8.

Plant GT, Hess RF, Thomas SJ. The pattern evoked electroretinogram in optic neuritis. Brain 1986; 109:469-90.

Potts AM, Inoue J. The electrically evoked response of the visual system (EER). Invest Ophthalmol Vis Sci 1968;7:269-78.

Potts AM, Inoue J. The electrically evoked response of the visual system (EER), Part 2 Effect of adaptation and retinitis pigmentosa. Invest Ophthalmol Vis Sci 1969;8:605-12.

Potts AM, Inoue J. The electrically evoked response of the visual system (EER), Part 3 Further contribution to the origin of the EER. Inves Ophthalmol Vis Sci 1970;9:814-819.

Riemslag FCC, Ringo JL, Spekreijse H, Verduin Lunel HF. The luminance origin on the pattern ERG in man. J Physiol 1985; 363:191.

Riggs LA, Johnson EP, Schick AM. Electrical responses of the human eye to moving stimulus patterns. Science 1964; 144:567-8.

Ringo J, Dijk BV, Spekreijse H. Pattern ERG of the cat. Vis Res. 1984; 24: 859-65.

Sandberg MA, Berson EL, Ariel M. Visually evoked response testing with a Stimular-ophthalmoscope. Arch Ophthalmol 1977; 95:1805-8.

Sandberg MA, Jacobson SG, Berson EL. Foveal cone electroretinograms in retinitis pigmentosa and juvenile macular degeneration. Am J Ophthalmol 1979; 88:702-7.

Sawusch M, Pokorny J, Smith VC. Clinical electroretinography for short wavelength sensitive cones. Invest Ophthalmol Vis Sci 1987;28:966-74.

Seiple WH, Kupersmith MJ, Nelson JI, Carr RE. The assessment of evoked potential contrast thresholds using real-time retrieval Invest Ophthalmol Vis Sci 1984; 25: 627-31.

Seiple WH, Siegel IM, Carr RE, Mayron C. Objective Assessment of temporal modulation transfer functions using the focal ERG. Am J Optom Physiol Opt 1986a; 63:1-6.

Seiple WH, Siegel IR, Carr RE, Mayron C. Evaluating Macular Function using the Focal ERG. Invest Ophthalmol Vis Sci 1986b; 27:1123-30.

Sherman J. Simultaneous pattern-reversal electroretinograms and visual evoked potentials in diseases of the macula and optic nerve. Ann NY Acad Sci 1982; 338: 214-25.

Shipley T. The visually evoked occipitogram in strabismic amblyopia under direct-view ophthalmoscopy. J Pediatric Ophthalmol 1969; 6:97-112.

Sieving PA, Steinberg RH. Contribution from proximal retina to intraretinal pattern ERG: the m-wave. Invest Ophthalmol Vis Sci 1985; 26: 1642-1647.

Skoog K. The c-wave of the human D.C. registered ERG III. Effects of ethyl alcohol on the c-wave. Acta Ophthalmol 1974;52:913-923.

Skoog K, Nilsson SEG. The c-wave of the Human DC registered ERG I. A Quantitative study of the relationship between c-Wave amplitude and Stimulus Intensity. Acta Ophthalmol 1974;52:759-773.

Spekreijse H, Estevez O, Van der Tweel LH Luminace responses to pattern reversal. Doc Ophthalmol Proc Ser 1973; 10: 205-11.

Steinberg RH. Interactions between the retinal pigment epithelium and the neural retina. Doc Ophthalmol 1985;60:327-46.

Steinberg RH, Miller SS. Aspects of elctrolyte transport in frog epithelium. Exp Eye Res 1973; 16: 365-72.

Steinberg RH, Linsenmeier RA, Griff ER. Retinal pigment epithelial cell contributions to the electroretinogram and electrooculogram. Prog in Retin Res 1985;4:33-66.

Sugimachi Y. MTF and VEP by laser interference fringes and its clinical use in ophthalmology. Proc 16th ISCV Symp, Morioka 1979:pp. 241-8.

Tamai M, Mizuno K. Electroretingram changes after fluorescein injection: a new method to evaluate blood-retinal barrier dysfunction. Invest Ophthalmol Vis Sci 1981; 20: 272-6.

Taumer R, Rohde N, Wichmann W, Rover JA. Method for DC-ERG Recording of Alert Humans. Albrecht Von Graefes Arch Klin Exp Ophthalmol 1976a;198:45-55.

Taumer R, Rohde N, Wichmann W., Rover J. Experiments Concerning the Human C-Wave. Albrecht Von Graefes Arch Klin. Exp Ophthalmol 1976b;198:139-53.

Taumer R, Wichmann W, Rohde N, Rover J. ERG of Humans without C-Wave. Albrecht Von Graefes Arch Klin Exp Ophthalmol 1976c;198:275-89.

Textorius O. The C-wave of the human electroretinogram in central retinal artery occlusion. Acta Ophthalmol 1978;56:827-36.

Textorius O, Nilsson SEG, Skoog K. Studies on acute and late stages of experimental central retinal artery occlusion in the cynomolgus monkey. Part 1:Intensity-amplitude relations of the D.C. recorded ERG with special reference of the C-wave. Acta Ophthalmol 1978;56:648-64.

Trick GL. PRRP. Abnormalities in glaucoma and ocular hypertension. Invest Ophthalmol Vis Sci 1986; 27: 1730-6.

Trick GL, Trick LR, Heywood KM. Altered pattern evoked retinal and cortical potentials associated with human senescence. Curr Eye Res 1986; 5:717-24.

Troelstra A, Schweitzer NMJ. Nonlinear analysis of the electroretinographic b-wave in man. J Neurophysiol 1968; 31: 588-606.

Tyler CW, Apkarian P, Levi DM, Nakayama K. Rapid assessment of visual function: an electronic sweep tchnique for the pattern visual evoked potential. Invest Ophthalmol Vis Sci 1979; 18: 703-13.

Vaegan, Billson FA. The differential effect of optic nerve disease on pattern and focal electroretinograms. Doc Ophthalmol 1987; 65: 45-56.

Vaegan, Billson FA. Macular electroretinograms and contrast sensitivity as sensitive detectors of early maculopathy. Doc Ophthalmol 1986; 63:399-406.

Vaegan, Billson F, Kemp S, Morgan M, Donnelley M, Montgomery P. Mavular electroretinograms: Their accuracy, specificity and implementation for clinical use. Aust J Ophthalmol 1984; 12:359-72.

Wanger P, Persson HE. Pattern reversal electroretinograms in unilateral glaucoma. Invest Ophthalmol Vis Sci 1983; 24: 749-53.

Wirth A. Beitrage zu den teilstromen des menschlichen elektoretinogramms. Albrecht Von Graefes Arch Klin Exp Ophthalmol 1974; 151: 662-71.

Wright KW, Eriksen JK, Shors TJ, Ary JP. Recording pattern visual evoked potentials under chloral hydrate sedation. Arch Ophthalmol 1986; 104: 718-21.

Yonemura D, Kawasaki K. New approaches to ophthalmic electrodiagnosis by retinal oscillatory potiential, drug-induced responses from retinal pigment epithelium and cone potential. Doc Ophthalmol 1979; 48: 163-222.

Yonemura J, Ishisaka J. On the elctrical excitability of the eye in congential achromatopsia. Tohoku J Exp Med 1955; 62; 377-89.

Chapter 6

Examination of the Ten Degrees of Visual field Surrounding Fixation

Michael Wall

Introduction

Of the 1.2 million retinal ganglion cell axons in the optic nerve, approximately 39% subserve the ten degrees of visual field surrounding fixation (central 10°) (Schein and de Monasterio, 1987). In spite of the importance of this area, when visual testing is performed, the central and paracentral areas are often neglected. In this chapter the various methods available for testing the 10° of visual field surrounding fixation are reviewed. Amsler grid testing is emphasized, as it is the most commonly used of these tests.

Historical Background and Literature Review

Albrecht von Graefe introduced visual field testing into clinical ophthalmology in 1856. He used a 3 x 4 ft blackboard divided into 3-in. squares as his campimeter and a piece of chalk as his test target (Fig. 6.1) (von Graefe, 1856). Jannik Peterson Bjerrum developed the Bjerrum screen in 1889 (Bjerrum, 1889). Using a test distance of 2 m and test objects as small as 1 mm, he was able to map accurately the central 10° (Fig. 6.2).

The tangent screen has largely been replaced by differential light-sensitivity bowl perimeters. This occurred because of superior reproduction of testing conditions and because the standardized, controlled test stimuli of the bowl perimeter allowed better quantitation. In addition, there was improved testing of the field of vision outside 30°. However, because of the prominent magnification effect when performed at 2 or 3 m, tangent screen examination is an excellent test for detection of scotomas in the central 10°.

With the widespread use of the Goldmann perimeter, following its introduction in 1945, there was improved quantitation of the visual sensitivity of the peripheral field. However, in many perimetrists' hands, there was a deemphasis of detailed testing of the central 10°. Testing of the central 10° is limited with the Goldmann device because the fixation monitor obstructs the central 2°. Therefore, adequate threshold testing requires use of the attachment for static perimetry. This device is expensive and cumbersome for routine use. In addition, testing of the central 10° is limited with the Goldmann perimeter because of the minifying effect of a short testing distance (30 cm). Although the Goldmann perimeter is an excellent apparatus for quantitation of the visual field, its main use is in testing the visual field outside the central 10°.

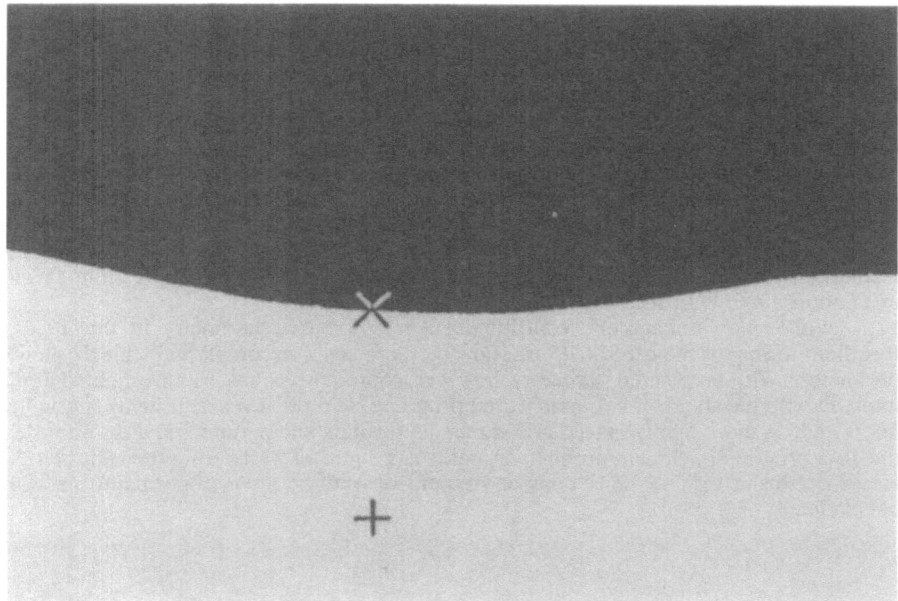

Figure 6.1. A first documented attempt at perimetry, von Graefe's "blackboard" campimeter. Note the superior altitudinal defect (from Von Graefe, 1856).

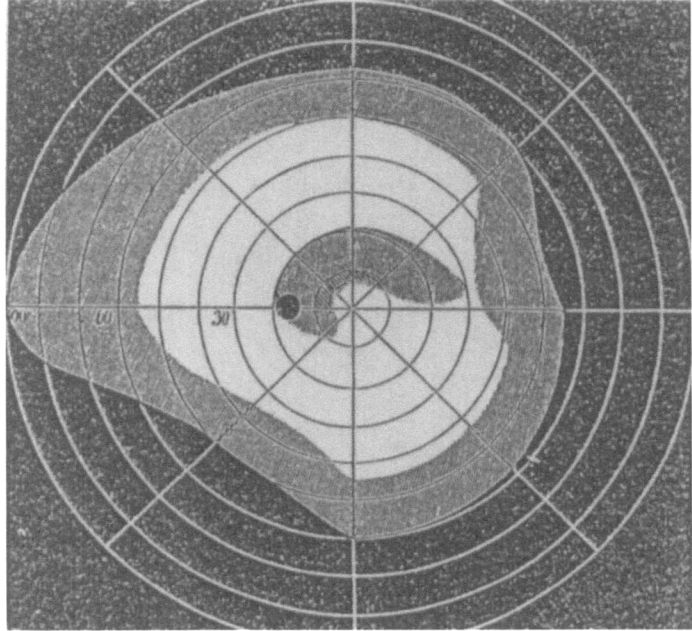

Figure 6.2. Bjerrum's attempt at quantitation of the visual field. Note the superior arcuate defect in a figure from Bjerrum's original paper (from Bjerrum, 1889).

Mark Amsler began development of a series of charts in the 1920s. They were designed specifically to qualitatively analyze the disturbances of visual function in the central 10° that accompanies the beginning and evolution of maculopathies. The charts were published by the Hamblin Company in 1949 and have since become standard equipment in ophthalmologist's offices (Amsler, 1947; Amsler, 1949; Amsler, 1953).

Amsler grid testing is an inexpensive and rapidly performed test. It employs a suprathreshold target to test the central 10°. It is excellent for detecting metamorphopsia, but is not sensitive for scotoma detection (Wall and Sadun, 1986).

Using cross-polarizing filters to vary perceived luminance (threshold Amsler grid testing), this test can be made more sensitive for finding scotomas and depressions (Wall and Sadun, 1986; Wall and May, 1987).

Following Fankhauser's contributions on automated perimetry in the 1970s, threshold testing of the central 10° can now be more easily accomplished with the bowl perimeter. With automated perimetry, however, coordinate points are thresholded at 6° intervals with the standard commonly used programs, and the foveal sensitivity is usually not tested. A more tightly spaced grid can be used with some perimeters. For example, the 10-2 program of the Humphrey perimeter has a grid of 2° covering the central 10°. However, this test is time consuming and expensive, and the limits of normality are still not evident.

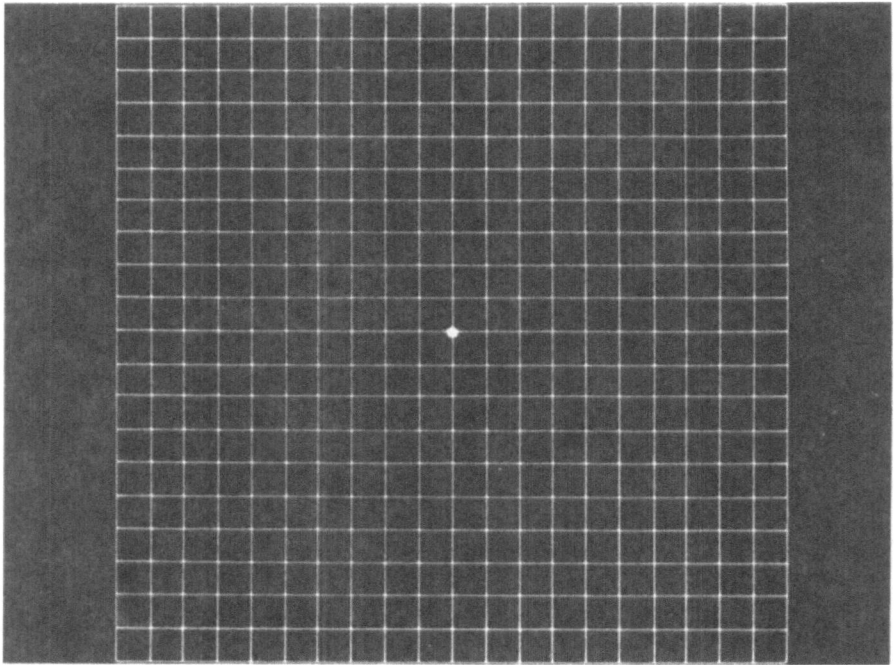

Figure 6.3: Standard white Amsler grid.

Recent Studies

Threshold Amsler grid testing is a technique used to increase the yield of scotoma detection in the central 10°. Using a device developed for brightness-sense testing by

Sadun and Lessell, which uses two cross-polarizing filters, the luminance of the target can be controlled (Fig. 2.2a,b) (Sadun and Lessell, 1985; Mainster and Dieckert, 1980). Subjects can then be asked to view the target with the grid being barely perceptible, i.e., at the threshold of detection (simulated in Fig. 6.3 and 6.4). Using this technique investigators have found the test to be much more sensitive for detecting shallow scotomas in patients with optic neuropathies and maculopathies (Wall and Sadun, 1986; Wall and May, 1987).

Figure 6.4: Simulation of threshold Amsler grid (from Wall and May, 1987).

Threshold Amsler grid testing is performed as follows: (1) The eye not being tested is occluded; (2) the patient is given the proper correction for near; (3) the standard white Amsler grid, (chart #1 in the Amsler Charts Manual with a white grid on black background) is held 28 to 30 cm from the eye; (4) the front polarizer is rotated so that the angle of polarization is slowly increased until the patient can barely see the white dot in the center of the grid but cannot see the grid (this is usually between 85° and 89° of polarization); (5) the angle of polarization is then slowly decreased 1° at a time until the grid can barely be seen (usually after 1° and 2°); this angle is recorded for reproduction of testing conditions at a follow-up office visit; (6) the patient views the target for no longer than several seconds (images in the periphery fade from view with prolonged viewing -- the Troxler effect); (7) the patient then draws any defects present. Since normal subjects may note that corners of the grid are missing, these defects are ignored. The black grid on white background should be used for patient drawings, not for testing.

Optic Neuropathies

Ten consecutive patients with optic neuropathies were studied to compare testing with 2-m tangent screen, automated perimetry, and Amsler grids (Wall and Sadun, 1986). Both standard white Amsler grid and threshold Amsler grid testing were performed. The screening strategy used for 2-m tangent screen examination is shown in Figure 6.5. The central 10° was surveyed with three different kinetic targets. The targets were chosen to produce isopters at 2.5°, 5°, and 10°. At times it was necessary to use a 1/2 mm red target to obtain a small enough isopter. Detection sensitivity was greatly enhanced by the incorporation of suprathreshold static tangent screen examination (Wall and Sadun, 1986). A static target was briefly presented 2° to 3° inside the equivalent kinetic stimulus. Since static images distant from fixation fade after several seconds (the Troxler effect), stimulus presentation time was brief. This technique was more sensitive for scotoma detection than kinetic tangent screen examination and autom. ed perimetry with 6° or 3° spaced grids (Wall and Sadun, 1986). The results of the study are shown in Figure 6.6.

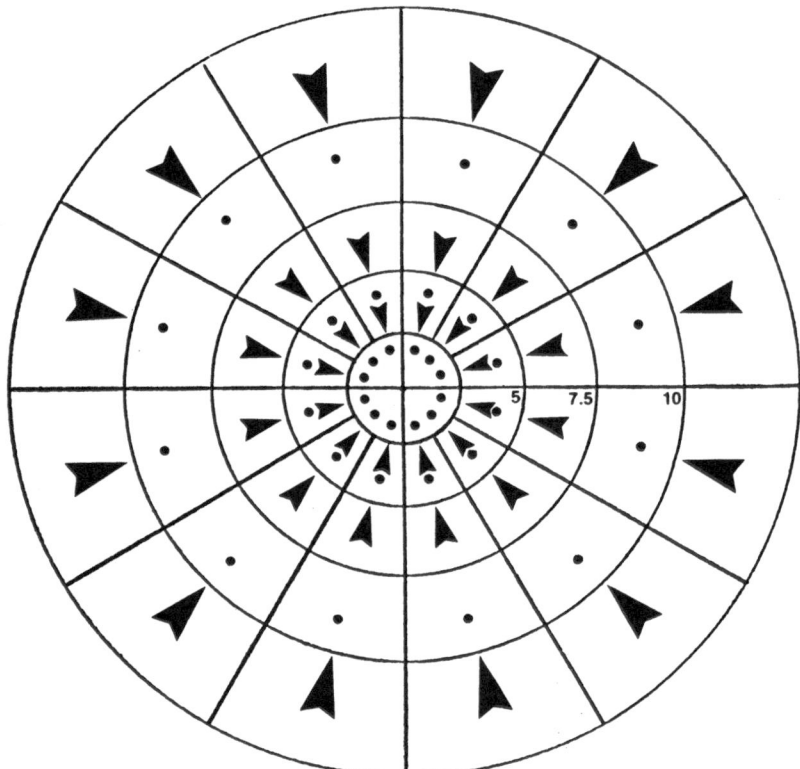

Figure 6.5. Screening strategy used for kinetic and static tangent screen examinations. Note the static targets (dots) are several degrees inside the corresponding kinetic target (arrowheads) (from Wall and Sadun, Arch Ophthalmol 104:520-23;1986 AMA).

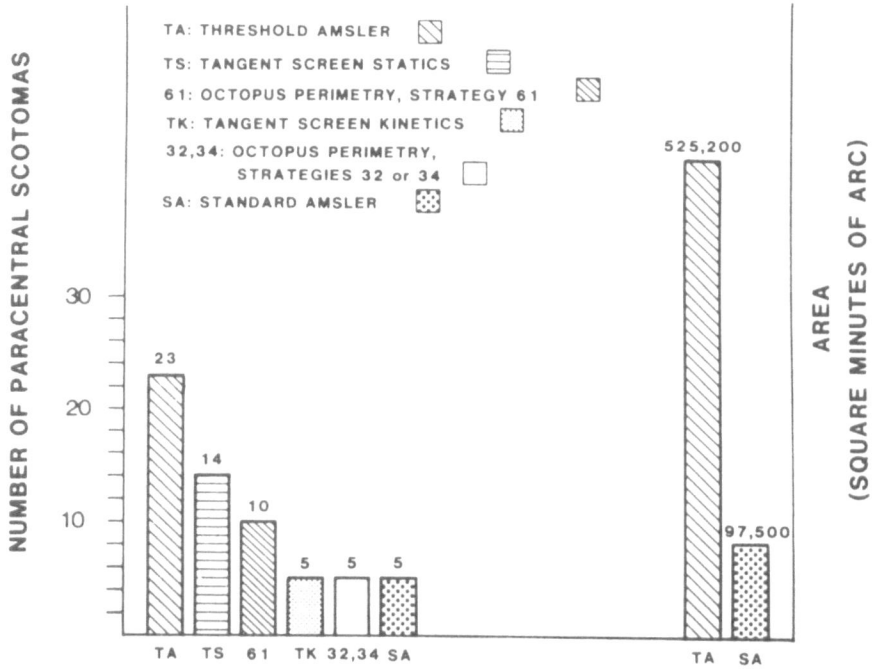

Figure 6.6. Comparisons of yields of visual screening methods used in 10 patients with optic neuropathies (from Wall and Sadun, Arch Ophthalmol 104:520-23;1986 AMA).

In this study, two-thirds of the defects found with threshold Amsler testing were confirmed with tangent screen or automated perimetry. Both the number of defects found and the total area of defects increased by a factor of 5 using threshold Amsler grid testing compared with standard white Amsler grid testing. Threshold Amsler grid testing was the most sensitive method of those used in the study.

Maculopathies

Threshold Amsler grid testing in maculopathies was studied in 10 patients who had normal standard white Amsler grid testing (Wall and May, 1987). All patients had ophthalmoscopic evidence of a macular lesion. The patients underwent a series of three additional Amsler grid tests. They were asked to view the following: (1) a red Amsler grid from the newest sets published by the Hamblin company, (2) a red grid from the older sets in which the lines are finer and less intense, and (3) a threshold Amsler grid, i.e., through cross-polarizing filters. The tests were each performed once during an office visit.

Following this, the patients had a three isopter kinetic and static tangent screen examination performed at 2 m to assess the central 10° of the visual field. The defects found with the various types of Amsler grid testing were specifically looked for with both kinetic and static tangent screen examinations.

Each patient underwent fundus photography. Fluorescein angiography was performed on eight of the 10 patients. Tables 6.1 and 6.2 show the results of this testing.

Table 6.1. Number of defects found with different
tests in patients with maculopathies

Test	No. of Defects
Standard Amsler grid	0
Bright red grid	1
Fine red grid	5
Threshold Amsler grid	12
Tangent screen	10
Confrontation visual fields	3

Table 6.2. Total area of defects in square minutes of arc
in patients with maculopathies

Test	Total
Standard Amsler grid	0
Bright red grid	4
Fine red grid	254
Threshold Amsler grid	527.5

It was found that metamorphopsia resolved as one progressed in the sequence of standard white grid, to the bright red grid, to fine red grid and lastly to the threshold Amsler grid.   With threshold Amsler grid testing, the area that had shown metamorphopsia was often the site of a field defect.

Threshold Amsler Grid Testing in Diabetics

Four different Amsler grid tests were used on 17 patients (30 eyes) with diabetes to determine whether alternate types of Amsler grid testing were of use in detecting visual loss in these patients.   As in the study on maculopathies, the grids used were the standard white Amsler grid, the bright red Amsler grid, the fine red Amsler grid, and the threshold Amsler grid using cross-polarizing lenses.

The total area of the scotomas found increased with decreasing grid intensity. Threshold Amsler grid testing was the most sensitive test (Table 6.3). In addition, as in the previous study (Wall and May, 1987), metamorphopsia resolved as grid intensity decreased (standard white Amsler grid most sensitive for metamorphopsia).   An example is shown in Figure 6.5. Six scotomas were detected with the standard white

Table 6.3. Results of Amsler grid testing
in patients with diabetes

Eye	DR grade	WA	BrRA	FRA	TA	Macula	Acuity
OD	no BDR	0	0	15	25	DMR	20/20
OS	no BDR	0	0	13	45	DMR	20/20
OD	no BDR	0	0	0	0	mac. edema	20/20
OS	no BDR	0	0	0	90	mac. edema	20/20
OD	mild BDR	0	0	24	34	normal	20/50
OS	mild BDR	0 M	0 M	46 M	46	normal	20/70
OD	no BDR	16	43	70	0	normal	20/20
OS	no BDR	0	0	0	0	normal	20/30
OD	mod BDR	122 M	161	237	237	macular exudate	20/50
OS	-	-	-	-	-	-	NLP
OD	-	-	-	-	-	-	CF
OS	pre-prol	0	0	0	0	DMR	20/30
OD	no BDR	0	0	0	19	DMR	20/30
OS	no BDR	0	0	0	100	DMR	20/25
OD	no BDR	0	0	0	0	normal	20/20
OS	no BDR	0	0	19	19	normal	20/20
OD	no BDR	40 M	120 M	180 M	180 M	DMR	20/20
OS	mild BDR	0 M	80 M	0 M	400 M	DMR	20/20
OD	no BDR	0	0	40	40	normal	20/20
OS	no BDR	0	0	29	29	normal	20/20
OD	no BDR	400	400	400	0	normal	20/20
OS	no BDR	400	400	400	400	normal	20/20
OD	no BDR	7	7	8	31	DMR	20/20
OS	no BDR	4	6	7	16	DMR	20/20
OD	mod BDR	0	90	23	89	mac. edema	20/50
OS	mod BDR	0	0	17	45	mac. edema	20/40
OD	no BDR	0	45	180	180	normal	20/80
OS	no BDR	-	-	-	-	COAG	20/400
OD	no BDR	60 M	20 M	56 M	400	DMR	20/20
OS	no BDR	0	0	0	0	DMR	20/20
OD	cataract	-	-	-	-	-	20/50
OS	no BDR	0	0	0	50	DMR	20/40
OD	no BDR	0	0	0	140	DMR	20/30
OS	no BDR	0	0	0	110	DMR	20/30
	Total	1,049	1,372	1,764	2,725		

OD = right eye, OS = left eye, DMR = decreased macular reflex, DR = diabetic retinopathy, BDR - background diabetic retinopathy, WA = standard white grid, BrRA = bright red grid, FRA = fine red grid, TA = threshold grid, COAG = chronic open angle glaucoma, NLP = no light perception, M = metemorphopsia.

Amsler grid; use of the bright red revealed 9; the fine red grid, 18. Scotomas were found with threshold Amsler grid testing in 23 of 30 (77%) of all eyes and in 16 of 24 (67%) of eyes without diabetic retinopathy.   Scotomas were found with fine red Amsler grid testing in 18 of 30 (60%) of all eyes and in 13 of 24 (54%) of eyes without diabetic retinopathy.

Discussion of Threshold Amsler Grid Testing

In these studies of threshold Amsler grid testing, comparison of the results of the test sequence from white Amsler to the bright red then to fine red and finally to the threshold grid showed a progressive increase in the number of scotomas detected and in the total area of the scotomas.   Use of the threshold stimulus in the optic neuropathy study increased the total scotoma area of 10 patients by approximately a factor of 5 (Wall and Sadun, 1986).   In addition, it has been shown that the defects found on threshold Amsler grid testing correlate with defects found with tangent screen and automated perimetry (Wall and Sadun, 1986; Wall and May, 1987).

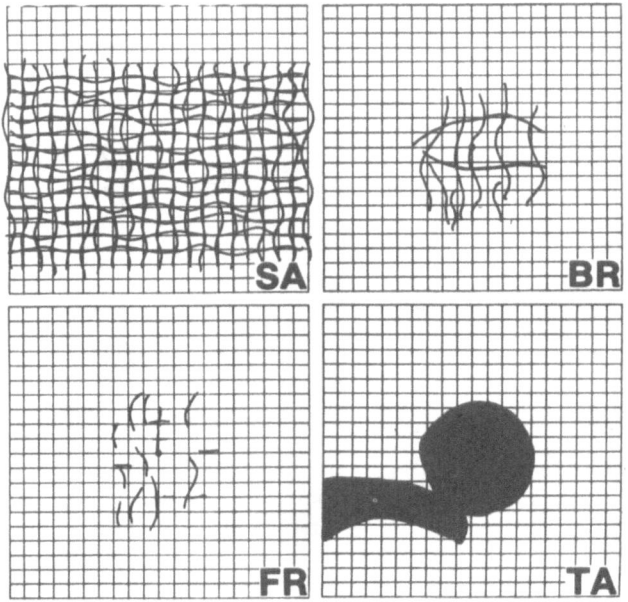

Figure 6.7.A: Note that the metamorphopsia decreases from standard Amsler grid testing (SA) to bright red grid testing (BR) to fine red grid testing (FR). Scotomas were observed faintly with the FR grid and easily with the threshold grid (TA).

Both threshold and standard Amsler grid testing may be sensitive tests, as Amsler grid testing may show metamorphopsia or scotomas when ophthalmoscopic examinations are normal (Amsler, 1949; Amsler, 1953).   In addition, Easterbrook has noted two patients with chloroquine retinopathy with relative scotomas on standard Amsler grid testing with normal color vision, electroretinograms, electro-oculograms, and fluorescein angiography (Easterbrook, 1984).   Conversely, patients with obvious macular abnormalities on funduscopic examination may not have defects present with standard Amsler grid testing (Wall and May, 1987). Of patients with maculopathies and normal standard white Amsler grid testing, most of these patients will have scotomas detectable if threshold Amsler grid testing is performed.

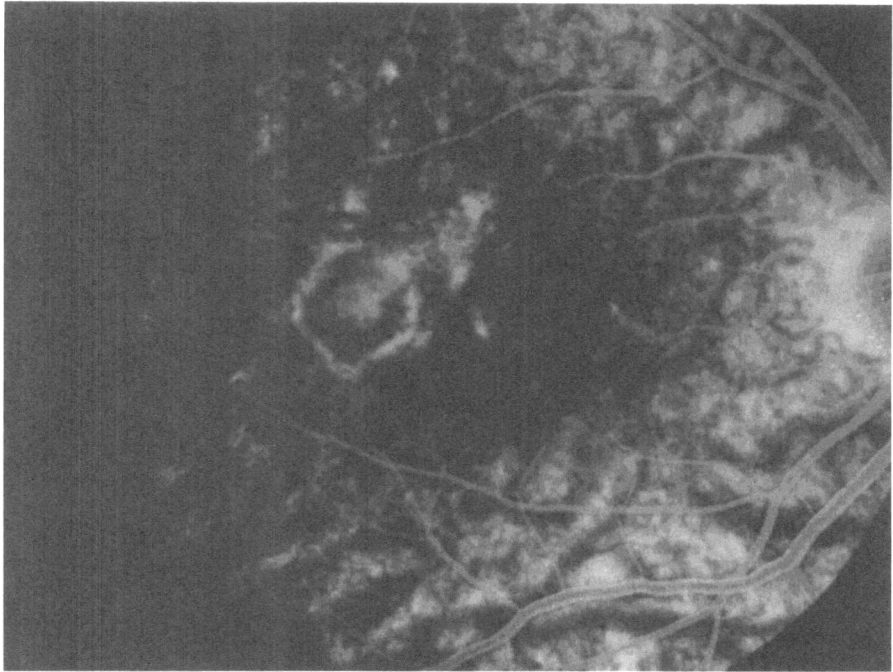

Figure 6.7 B: Fluorescein angiogram shows RPE dropout in the macula with a laser scar temporal and superior to the fovea (from Wall and May, 1987).

A limitation of these studies of threshold Amsler grid testing is that the examinations were only performed once. As with any new psychophysical test, intratest and intertest reproducibility must be demonstrated. The evidence that the defects found is real is that normal subjects miss only corners with threshold Amsler grid testing, and most of the scotomas found can be confirmed with another type of perimetry (Wall and Sadun, 1986; Wall and May, 1987; Matsuo et al, 1972).

It is known that suprathreshold perimetry strategies may fail to detect some relative scotomas. The Amsler grid is a suprathreshold target and is analogous to mapping the visual island with a perimetric stimulus of high luminance. Use of the threshold grid is analogous to surveying the central 10° with a low luminance target (Fig. 6.6). This is most likely the mechanism of the increased yield of visual field defects with threshold Amsler grid testing.

With threshold testing, the area that had previously produced metamorphopsia often becomes the site of a visual field defect, i.e., as the contrast of the grid on the background was decreased the patient's metamorphopsia resolved. Therefore, the standard white Amsler grid should be performed for metamorphopsia, and threshold Amsler grid for scotoma detection.

Other Types of Amsler Grid Testing

The Amsler grid has been modified for "dynamic " testing in which the grid is used as a background for tangent screen testing (Chen and Frenkel, 1975).   It has been transilluminated for visual testing in patients with cataracts (Miller et al, 1978; Bernth-Petersen, 1981).   This technique increased the illuminance of the grid, making it even more suprathreshold.   Using a scanning laser ophthalmoscope investigators have projected the grid on to patients' maculas (Mainster et al, 1982). A wallet-sized grid has been popularized by Yannuzzi (1982), and Frisén (1987) has included grids of various levels of intensity in his battery of personal computer visual testing programs.

Examples of Amsler grid testing

The Amsler grid is useful for detecting both metamorphopsia and scotomas.   The location and type of the metamorphopsia may suggest the pathology present.   For example, the central micropsia present in Figure 6.7 implies an increase in spacing between photoreceptors in the fovea.   Radial cecocentral metamorphopsia occurs with the photoreceptor elevation of disc edema (Fig. 6.8).

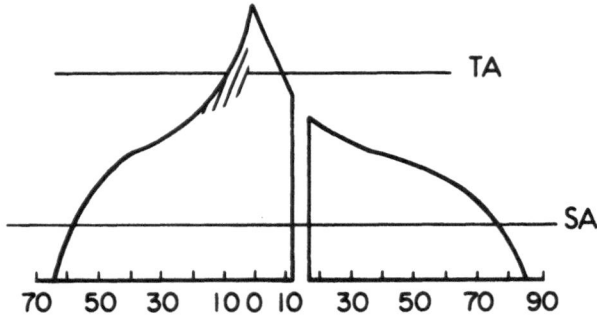

Figure 6.8. Sagittal section of visual island as would be plotted by static perimetry. Abscissa is degrees from central fixation. Ordinate is visual sensitivity. Relative scotoma (diagonal lines) is detected by threshold Amsler grid testing (TA). Standard Amsler grid (SA) stimulus surveys the island at too great a depth to detect the scotoma (from Wall and Sadun, Arch Ophthalmol 104:520-23;1986 AMA).

Multiple paracentral scotomas ("Swiss cheese" defect) are common in the optic neuropathy of multiple sclerosis (Fig. 6.9). Cecocentral defects may also be detected in various optic neuropathies (Fig. 6.10). Foveal disorders may produce central scotomas with or without metamorphopsia.   The sparing of foveal sensitivity with parafoveal depression in maculopathies as described by Hart (Hart, 1983; Hart et al, 1984) may be found with threshold Amsler grid testing (Fig. 6.11, hereditary dominant drusen). An example of how lesion position and shape can correlate with the defect is shown in Figure 6.12 in a case of presumed histoplasmosis. Bjerrum scotomas may be found with Amsler grid testing (Fig. 6.13). This example, found with a standard Amsler grid, was also present with threshold Amsler grid testing. However, since normal subjects may miss corners of the grid with threshold Amsler grid testing, the scotoma could not be designated.

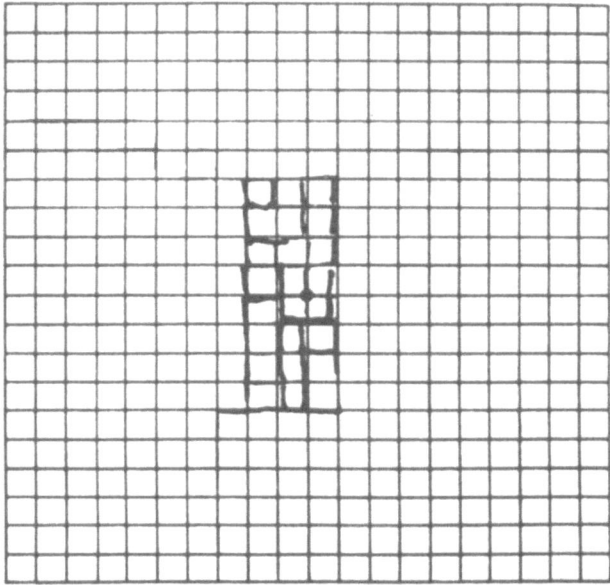

Figure 6.9. Micropsia of the central field indicates an increase in spacing between foveal photoreceptors.

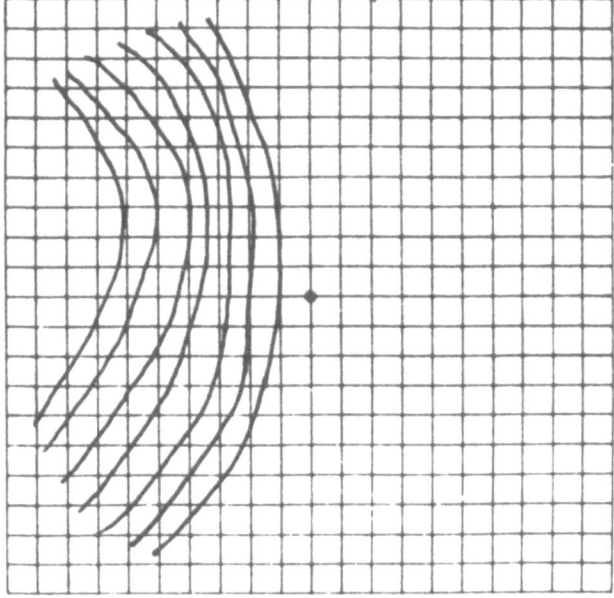

Figure 6.10. Cecocentral metamorphopsia of the left eye in a radial pattern occurs with the photoreceptor displacement of disc edema in a patient with pseudotumor cerebri.

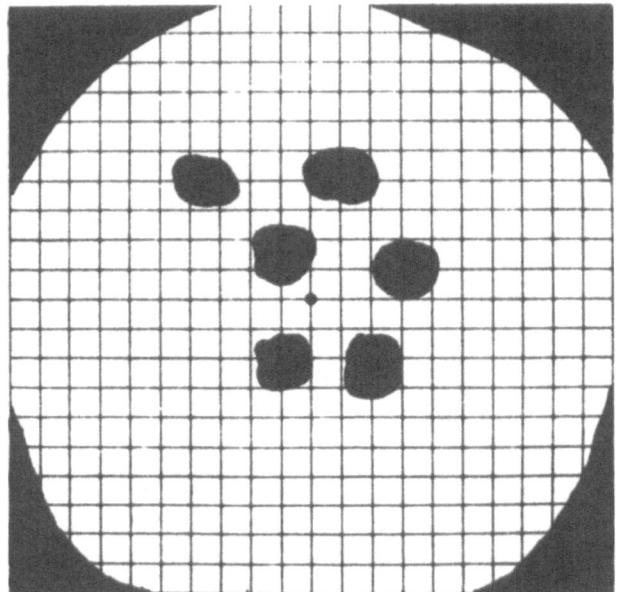

Figure 6.11. Multiple paracentral scotomas in optic neuritis.

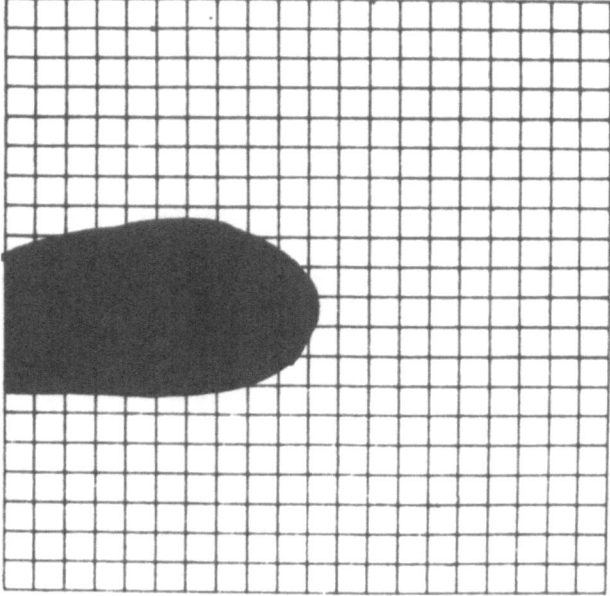

Figure 6.12. A typical cecocentral defect found in various optic neuropathies.

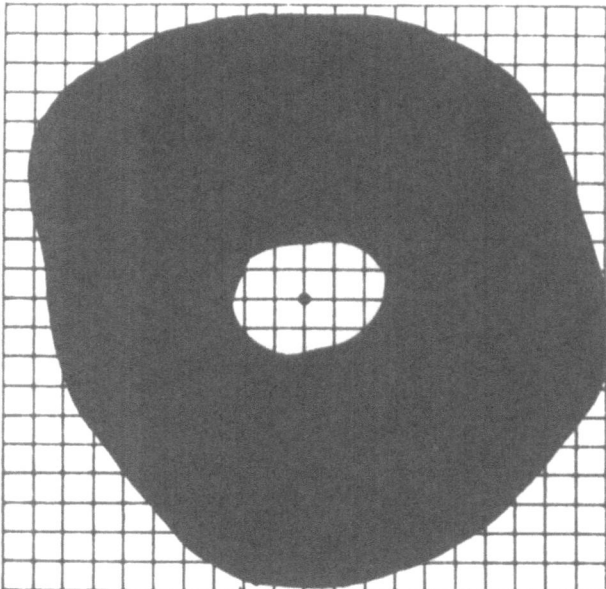

Figure 6.13.A: A patient with hereditary dominant drusen with sparing of foveal sensitivity associated with parafoveal depression found with threshold Amsler grid testing.

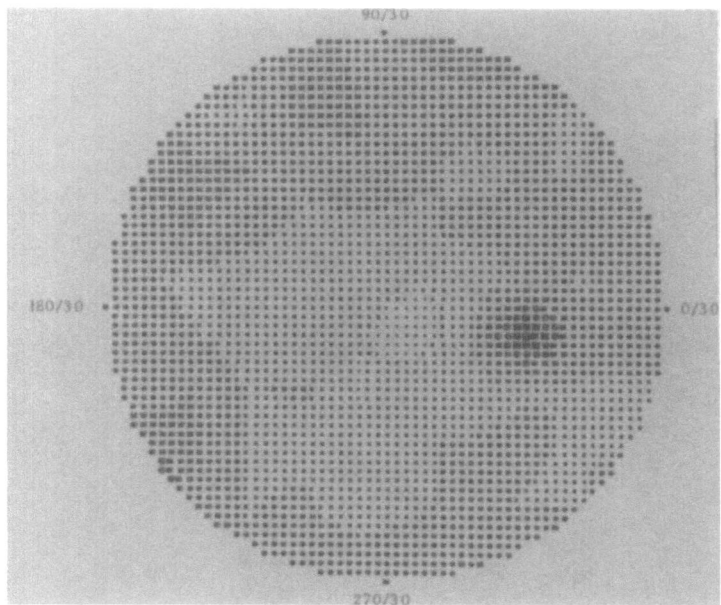

Figure 6.13.B: The automated visual field of the central 30° is normal in the central 10°.

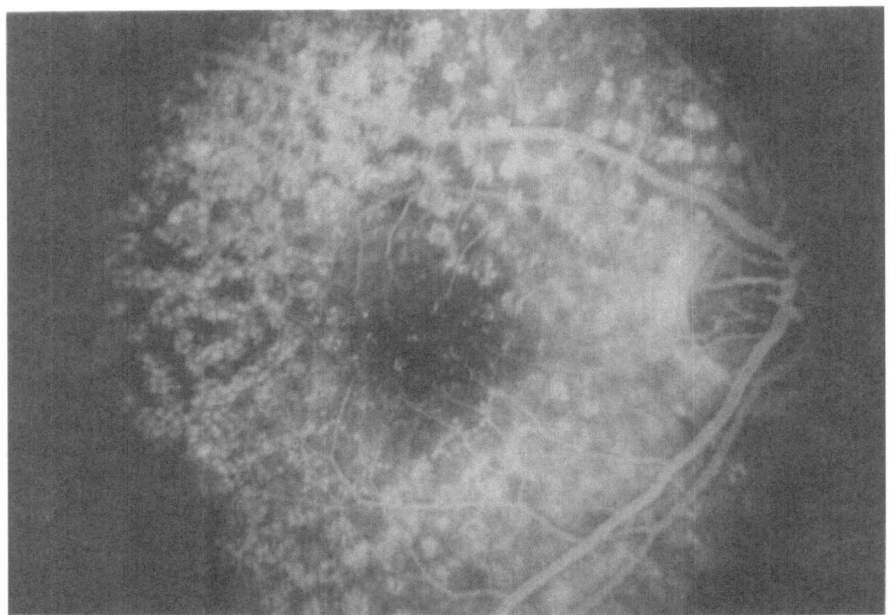

Figure 6.13.C: A fluorescein angiogram shows discrete window defects in the retinal pigment epithelium.

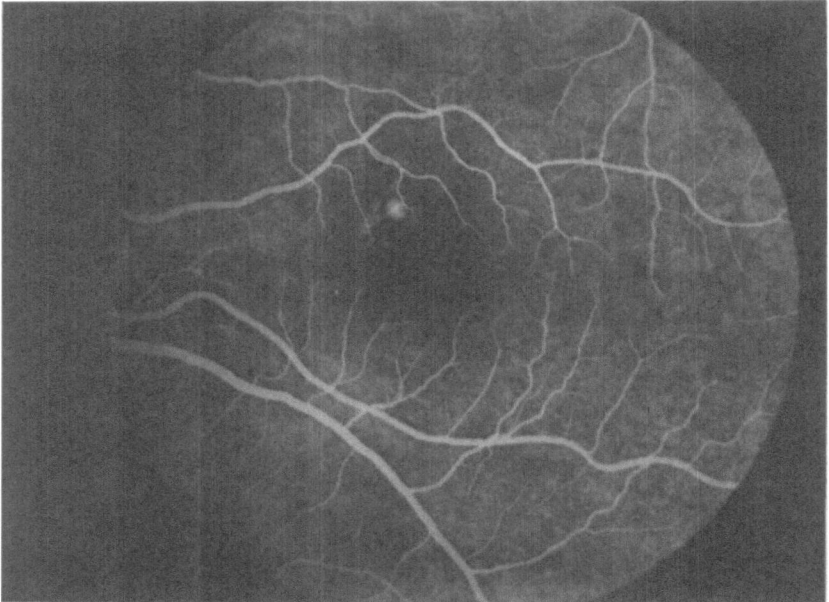

Figure 6.14.A: Note the RPE window defect present on the fluorescein angiogram in the superior nasal macula.

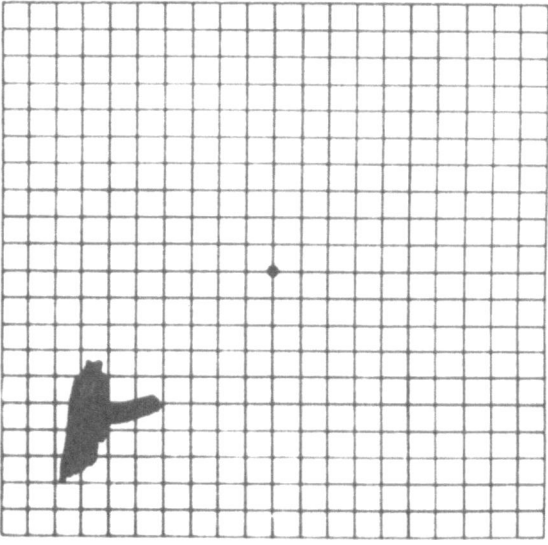

Figure 6.14.B: This corresponds to the inferotemporal defect present with threshold Amsler grid testing (from Wall and May, 1987).

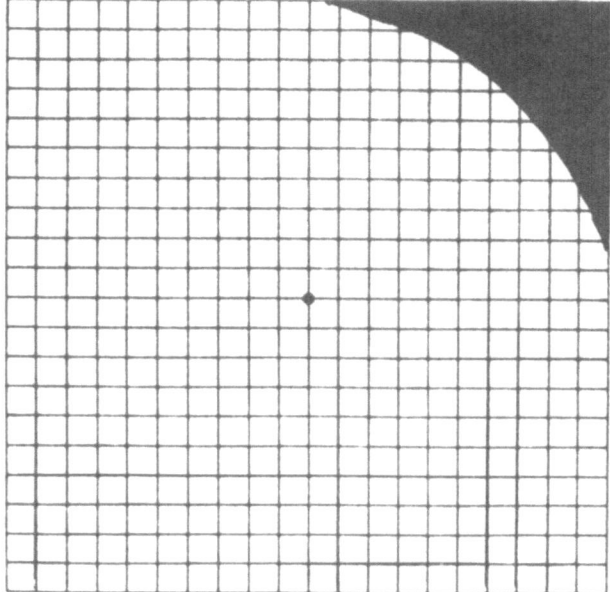

Figure 6.15. A superior Bjerrum scotoma in the right eye of a patient with pseudotumor cerebri found with the standard grid. Normal subjects may miss corners of the grid with the threshold test.

Automated Perimetry of the Central 10°

There has been little published on automated visual field testing of programs that evaluate the central 10°. Younge (1985) studied 62 patients with possible multiple sclerosis aged 18 to 39 using OCTOPUS program #11. This program tests the foveal threshold and the 3° surrounding fixation with a 3° grid. A total of 61% of the patients with definite multiple sclerosis had abnormal testing, 54% of the patients with possible multiple sclerosis had abnormal testing, and 33% of patients without multiple sclerosis had abnormal automated perimetry. Seventeen patients had abnormal automated perimetry with a normal visual evoked response. However, 17 patients also had an abnormal visual evoked response with normal automated perimetry.

Brusini and colleagues (1987) developed a strategy for testing the cecocentral area to test chronic alcoholics. Thirty-nine percent of the patients had visual loss in this area in one or both eyes.

Rolando and associates (1987) studied the foveal threshold and the central 10° along the vertical and horizontal meridians in patients with glaucoma. They found a significant difference in mean sensitivity in this area during periods of high pressure and lower pressure.

It is likely that programs of the central 10° (like the 2° spaced grid of the 10-2 program of the central 10° of the Humphrey automated perimeter) will be useful for various toxic and other optic neuropathies.

Future of the Tests

We foresee the use of threshold Amsler grid testing not only in the detection of visual loss but also in the follow-up evaluation of patients. For example, patients predisposed to subretinal pigment epithelial neovascular membrane formation or those taking potentially toxic agents such as chloroquine might benefit from serial threshold Amsler grid testing.

With faster and more sensitive perimetric strategies, e.g., high-pass resolution perimetry, evaluation of the central 10° should improve. Hopefully, more attention will be paid to the central 10° in future test development.

Summary

Although the central 10° of the visual field is an area of vital importance, it is often not thoroughly tested with commonly used strategies. Threshold Amsler grid testing is a rapid and sensitive technique for the evaluation of the central 10° of visual field in patients with maculopathies and optic neuropathies. Both standard white Amsler grid testing (for metamorphopsia) and threshold testing (for visual field defects) can be performed for general sensory visual screening. Automated perimetry strategies for the central 10° are gaining in popularity. They are limited by the long testing time and determination of limits of normality. One hopes that new testing strategies will emphasize testing of this important area.

References

Amsler M. Earliest symptoms of disease of the macula. Br J Ophthalmol 1953;37:521-37.

Amsler M. L'examen qualitatif de la fonction maculaire. Ophthalmologica 1947;1142:248-61.

Amsler M. Quantitative and qualitative vision. Trans Ophthalmol Soc UK 1949;69:397-410.

Bernth-Petersen P. An evaluation of the transilluminated Amsler grid for macular testing in cataract patients. Acta Ophthalmol 1981;59:57-63.

Bjerrum JP. An addition to the general examination of the field of vision. Scand O Mag 1889;2:141-85.

Brusini P, Dal Mas P, Della Mia G. et al. Centro-cecal field examination in alcoholics. Doc Ophthalmol Proc Ser 1987;49:639-44.

Chen KFS, Frenkel M. Dynamic visual field testing using the Amsler grid patterns. Trans Am Acad Ophthalmol Otolaryngol 1975;79:OP761-OP71.

Easterbrook M. The use of Amsler grids in early chloroquine retinopathy. Ophthalmology 1984;91:1368-72.

Frisén L. A computer-graphics visual field screener using high-pass resolution targets and multiple feedback devices. Doc Ophthalmol Proc Ser 49, 1987;441-6.

Hart WM, Burde RM, Johnston GP, Drews RC. Static perimetry in chloroquine retinopathy. Perifoveal patterns of visual field depression. Arch Ophthalmol 1984;102:377-80.

Hart WM, Henkind P (ed). Three-dimensional topography of the central visual field: sparing of foveal sensitivity in macular disease. ACTA XXIV International Congress of Ophthalmology. J.B. Lippincott: 1983.

Mainster MA, Dieckert JP. A simple haploscopic method for quantitating color brightness comparison. Am J Ophthalmol 1980;89:58-61.

Mainster MA, Timberlake GT, Webb RH, et al. Scanning laser ophthalmoscopy: Clinical applications. Ophthalmology 1982;89:852-57.

Matsuo H, Ohta Y, Endo N, Kato H. Studies on the new central scotometric plates. Acta Soc Ophthalmol Jpn 1972;76:1336-43.

Miller D, Lamberts DW, Perry HD. An illuminated grid for macular testing. Arch Ophthalmol 1978;96:901-2.

Rolando M, Corallo G, Gandolfo E, Zingirein M. Glaucoma follow-up by means of central differential threshold measurements. Doc Ophthalmol Proc Ser 1987;49:407-11.

Sadun A, Lessell S. Brightness-sense and optic nerve disease. Arch Ophthalmol 1985;103:39-43.

Schein SJ, de Monasterio FM. Mapping of retinal and geniculate neurons onto striate cortex of macaque. J Neurosci 1987;7:996-1009.

Von Graefe A. Examination of the visual field in amblyopic disease. Arch Ophthalmol 1856;2:258-98.

Wall M, May DR. Threshold Amsler grid testing in maculopathies. Ophthalmology 1987;94:1126-33.

Wall M, Sadun AA. Threshold Amsler grid testing; cross-polarizing lenses enhance yield. Arch Ophthalmol 1986;104:520-23.

Yannuzzi L. A modified Amsler grid. Ophthalmology 1982;89:157-9.

Younge BR. Computerized perimetry in neuro-ophthalmology. In Spaeth GL, Whalen WR (eds) Computerized Visual Fields. Thorofare, New Jersey: Slack Inc: 1985; pp. 239-276.

Chapter 7

Automated Perimetry: Theoretical and Practical Considerations

Richard P. Mills

Introduction

The basis for perimetry as practiced in most clinical settings is the patient's ability to detect a spot of light against a uniform background illumination: so-called differential light sensitivity. The popularity of this testing methodology relates to the nearly universal ability of patients to understand the task expected of them, to apply a reasonably uniform criterion for responding to stimuli, and to demonstrate an age-specific range of normality that allows separation of abnormal results with acceptable, though by no means ideal, sensitivity and specificity. However, differential light sensitivity perimetry is a crude test and does not necessarily relate to the ways in which retinal sensitivity is arrayed. For example, more complex stimuli can be designed to maximally stimulate the receptive fields of certain classes of ganglion cells. Experience with more complex methodologies than differential light sensitivity has in the past demonstrated an unacceptable specificity (high false-positive rate) in the detection of abnormality. Nonetheless, some recent breakthroughs have occurred, and more may be expected as we attempt to detect disease at progressively earlier stages through psychophysical testing.

In the past decade a revolution in perimetry involving differential light sensitivity has occurred. Static methods of exploring the visual field have supplanted kinetic methods in routine clinical use. The principal reason for this dramatic shift in practice has been the availability of computerized perimeters, which are easier to program for static testing.

Historical Background and Literature Review

Kinetic perimetry

The tangent screen and the Goldmann perimeter are the time-honored devices for testing the visual field. Stimuli of various intensities are moved from the nonseeing periphery toward the center, and the patient responds when he or she detects the stimulus. The borderline between seeing and nonseeing can be drawn by connecting the points derived from a single stimulus strength, the familiar isopter of kinetic perimetry. If the chosen stimulus is quite weak, the isopter may form a circle around fixation inside the physiologic blind spot. If the stimulus is strong, the maximum field area is outlined

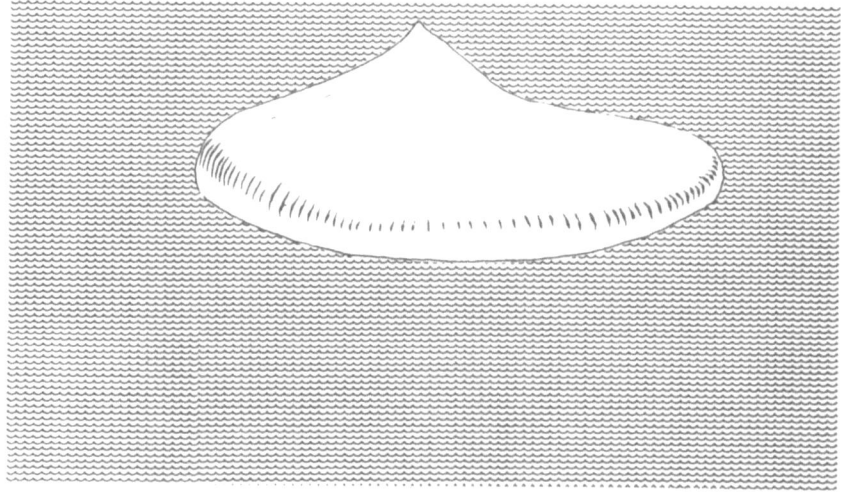

Figure 7.1. Traquair's island of vision in a sea of blindness. The highest point, representing the fovea, has the greatest sensitivity to test stimuli. At the water level the sensitivity is zero and no stimulus can be seen. The slope of the normal island of vision varies, being steepest close to the fovea and at the edge of the island, and more gentle in the intermediate sections.

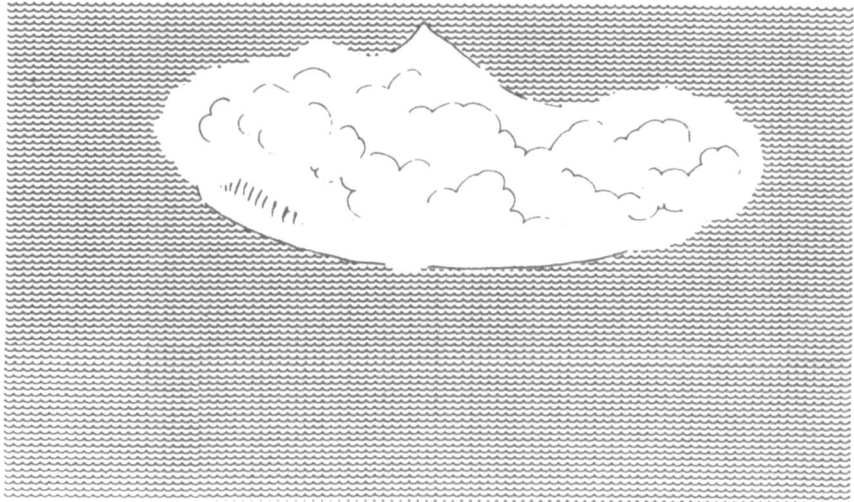

Figure 7.2. The problem in clinical perimetry is that the island of vision is enshrouded in fog and must be indirectly mapped. Note the peak is exposed, since we know something about it from visual acuity testing.

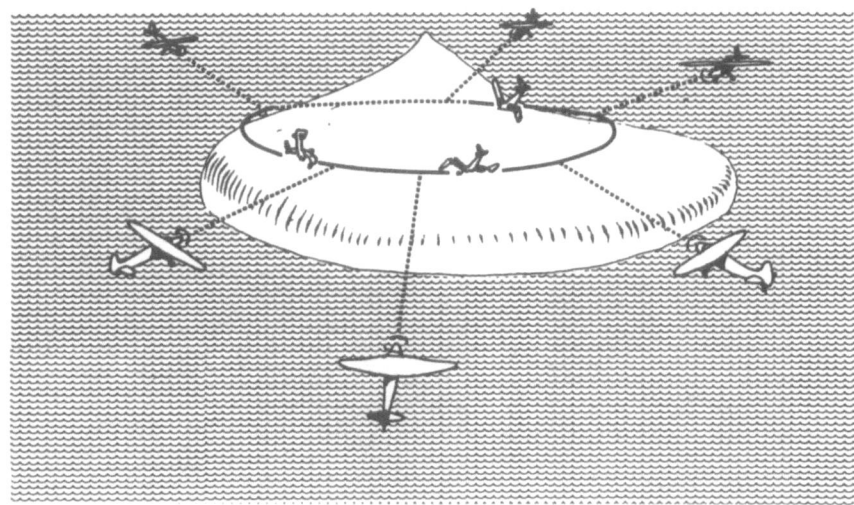

Figure 7.3. The island can be mapped by flying many airplanes toward it at the same altitude and recording where they crash. Knowing the altitude, we can draw various isopters and then have an idea of the slope of the hill of vision. This principle is used with the Goldmann instrument or tangent screen.

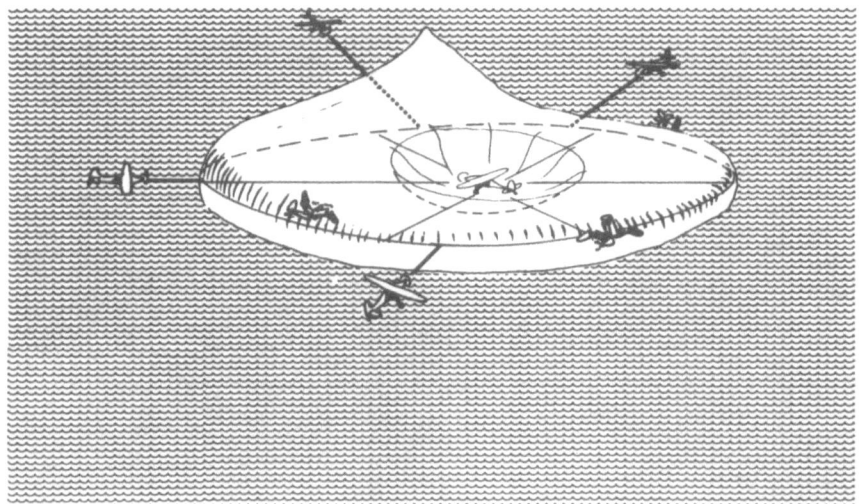

Figure 7.4. With kinetic perimetry depressions of the interior of the island of vision are easy to miss. The airplanes will all crash on the periphery of the island or fly over the depression to crash centrally. Only if we are lucky enough to start an airplane in the center of the depression will we discover its presence.

by the isopter at a perimeter, since the limits of testing at the tangent screen are exceeded.   An array of isopters can be plotted on a visual field chart, and ophthalmologists feel comfortable interpreting such charts.

It should be remembered that kinetic perimetry depends on a gradation of retinal sensitivity increasing from the periphery toward the center of the field, or from the center of a scotoma toward the surrounding area. Thus, a constant stimulus strength will be unseen on one side and seen on the other side of the isopter line. The location of the isopter line denotes the points at which the stimulus just reaches the threshold of perception. In order that we use a consistent method of approaching the threshold, and one that gives the most reproducible results, the stimulus in kinetic perimetry is always moved from nonseeing areas into seeing areas of the field.

Unfortunately, kinetic perimetry suffers from five disadvantages that limit its usefulness. To explain these disadvantages the old Traquair analogy of the island of vision in a sea of blindness (Traquair, 1927) can be recalled (Mills, 1984a) (Fig. 7.1).

The highest points on the island represent the best retinal sensitivity, where weak stimuli can be detected. Down near the waterline, only the strongest stimuli can be seen and sensitivity is poor. The hill is, of course, enshrouded in fog, and the job of the perimetrist is to map it (Fig. 7.2).

In kinetic perimetry, a stimulus of known strength is moved centrally, like an airplane flying toward the island at known altitude. The airplane "stimulus" will crash when it hits the island. After a number of airplane stimuli have crashed at one altitude, we can draw an isopter. After drawing several isopters, we will have a topographic map of the island of vision (Fig. 7.3).

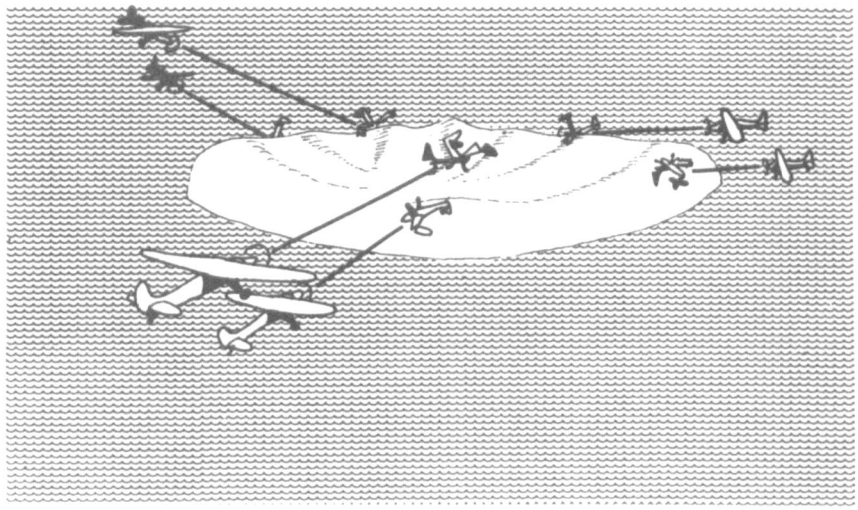

Figure 7.5. Another difficulty with kinetic perimetry is that flat sections of the island are difficult to map. Airplanes flying toward the island at one altitude may crash centrally, whereas those flying at a slightly different altitude will crash peripherally. Moreover, undulations of the flat section will be undiscovered.

The first of five disadvantages of kinetic perimetry is that depression in the interior of the island of vision is difficult to detect. Stimuli (airplanes) coming from the outside will miss it (Fig. 7.4).

We could start the stimulus within the depression, of course, if we knew it was there in advance. Since we usually do not, we would be forced to select places to start the stimulus randomly, hoping we would start inside a depression (scotoma). The chance of missing isolated depressions (scotomas) is high, especially with small or shallow ones.

The second disadvantage is that kinetic perimetry does a poor job of mapping flat sections of the island of vision. An airplane stimulus coming from outside at one altitude may crash quite a distance away from one coming at a slightly different altitude (Fig. 7.5).

Undulations of the flat section, which may be quite important, will be unmapped. Most patients have at least some relatively flat areas in their visual island, like a plateau, but in some patients the entire island resembles a mesa. In such patients, kinetic perimetry tends not to be a very productive exercise.

Third, kinetic perimetry by definition uses moving stimuli. It has long been known that moving stimuli are easier to detect than stimuli that are standing still, especially within defective areas of the visual field. One of the reasons for this is that more retinal ganglion cell receptive fields are stimulated by a moving target. Known as statokinetic dissociation (the Riddoch phenomenon), and contrary to popular belief, it occurs with lesions at all levels of the visual pathways, although it may be most prominent in occipital lobe disease. The fact that the stimulus is moving may cause a visual field defect to be missed.

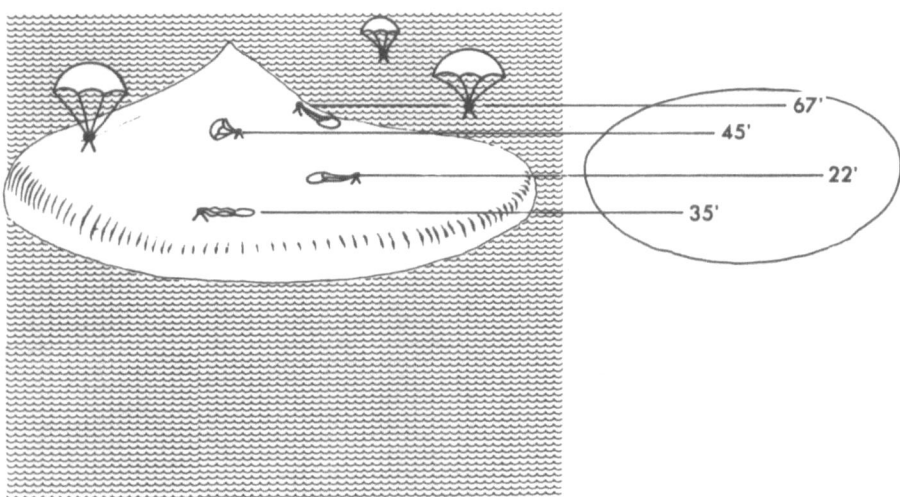

Figure 7.6. Another method of mapping the island of vision is to drop parachutes at known coordinates toward the island and record the height at which they land. The principle is the same for static threshold determinations in clinical perimetry. Although time consuming, we know all there is to know about each point and can map the island if we test enough points.

Fourth, the isopter maps generated by kinetic perimetry do not lend themselves easily to statistical analysis, as numeric data do. Since a visual field examination is a set of measurements in a biologic system and an exercise in probability, the results of testing should be suited to statistical analysis. Spatial data, presented on two dimensional maps that distort the hemispheric surface of the perimeter bowl, are statistically more difficult to analyze than a set of numbers.

Finally, kinetic perimetry has proved difficult to automate, except for simple testing of a peripheral isopter. Undue amounts of time are easily expended attempting to test relatively flat areas of the visual island, where the location of the isopter boundary may vary a great deal on multiple stimulus presentations, and the computer cannot reconcile the inconsistencies.

Before the appearance of automated perimeters, Armaly developed and Drance modified (Rock et al, 1971) a method of screening for glaucomatous field that lessened the effect of the first three disadvantages of kinetic perimetry. They did so by including in the test strategy a series of stimuli presented statically within the central visual field along with the kinetic peripheral isopters. This screening method was actually a mixture of kinetic and static test strategies.

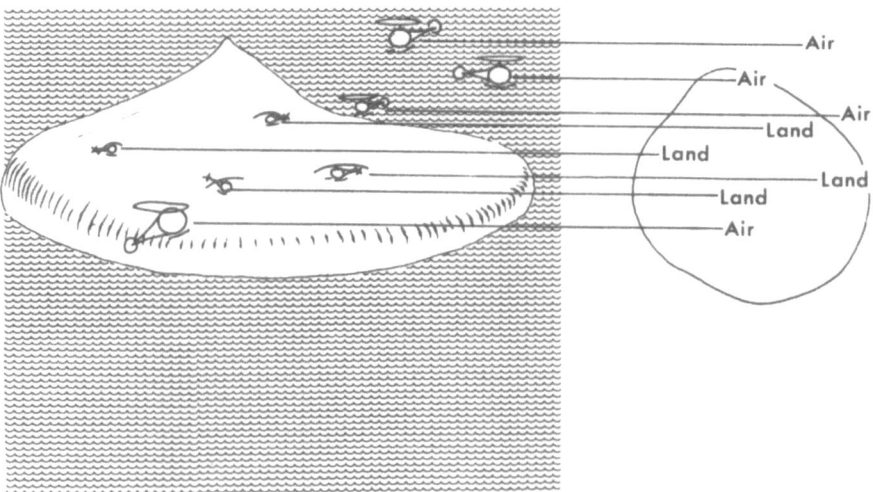

Figure 7.7. Another method of mapping the island of vision is to employ helicopters to fly to known coordinates and altitude and report simply whether they are in the air or have landed. The same principle applies for suprathreshold testing in clinical perimetry. A large number of points can be tested in a short time, but we know only whether each point is seen or not seen. With a sufficient variety of stimulus strengths, a map of the island of vision can be generated.

Static Perimetry

The clinical value of testing with nonmoving stimuli was first reported by Ferree et al (1933), but it was not until Harms and Aulhorn (1959) designed the Oculus (Tubinger) perimeter that the method gained wide acceptance.

Refer again to the island of vision analogy to see how static perimetry works. We could drop parachutes with altimeters onto the island and record the height at which each landed. Thus, at a number of discrete locations in space, we would know the height (sensitivity) (Fig. 7.6).

This method is known as threshold static perimetry, since it determines the threshold between seeing and nonseeing at a number of preselected locations. Static perimetry determines the unknown threshold stimulus value at a known point whereas kinetic perimetry determines the unknown point at which a known stimulus reaches threshold.

Threshold static perimetry overcomes many of the disadvantages of kinetic perimetry. Isolated depressions (scotomas) in the island of vision are less likely to be missed if one uses a high enough density of stimulus locations. Flat areas of the island are accurately defined, and undulations unmasked. The stimulus is not moving, the numeric data can easily be manipulated statistically, and the process is easy to computerize. Unfortunately, threshold determinations are quite time consuming, and long testing sessions are required to develop adequate point density. The reluctance of patients and perimetrists to commit to long testing sessions is a problem that becomes even worse if screening of significant patient numbers is desired. In addition, test reliability lessens in some subjects as the length of the examination increases.

To save testing time but retain some of the advantages of static perimetry, suprathreshold static testing methods were developed. Helicopters are employed to fly to certain locations over the island of vision and hover at a specified altitude. They indicate whether they are still in the air or whether they have landed (Fig. 7.7).

A large number of points in space at different altitudes can be tested in a relatively short time. If we select our points well, we can detect depressions of the interior of the island. We will still have difficulty mapping flat areas of the island and determining undulations of the surface, and the data are not suitable for statistical manipulation. But we are still using static stimuli, and automation of the process is simple.

One problem with suprathreshold static perimetry is that it is easy to waste considerable time testing with stimulus strengths that are either way above threshold or way below it. If we choose a single stimulus strength to test the entire field, it may be too strong centrally yet too weak peripherally because of the decreasing sensitivity with increasing eccentricity from the center. In fact, unless we select stimulus strengths that are just stronger than threshold at each location, we are likely to miss subtle scotomas.

If we only knew what the expected threshold between seeing and nonseeing was at any point on the island, we could select our stimulus strength close to the expected threshold. This would allow us to detect scotomas or depressions across the entire field because we would be using different stimulus strengths at different places in the field: weaker toward the center and stronger toward the outside.

To accomplish this, we could use a threshold static method at a few points in the field, determining the actual threshold at those points. We could then select stimuli for our suprathreshold test related to (interpolated from) those few threshold determinations. Such a strategy is called threshold-related suprathreshold static perimetry. Other threshold-related strategies might employ stimuli selected on the basis of age-corrected normal values at certain visual field locations, or might vary the stimulus strength with distance from fixation.

In summary, three types of static perimetry are commonly used in automated perimeters. Threshold static perimetry determines the threshold stimulus strength at specified locations in the field. Suprathreshold static perimetry presents a preselected stimulus at specified locations and determines whether it is seen or not. Threshold-related suprathreshold static perimetry presents stimuli at specified locations, with stimulus strength chosen on the basis of a few known threshold points or other information.

Automation of Perimetry

Full automation of the kinetic perimeter was an attractive goal that proved impossible to achieve. However, more success was achieved by groups working with static devices, most notably in Switzerland (Fankhauser, 1972) and Sweden (Heij and Krakau, 1975). As these groups and others grappled with the problem of programming a computer to test the visual field, they found the existing level of knowledge about the principles of light-sense perimetry to be inadequate. Accordingly, a series of investigations followed that established a range of desirable test parameters and strategies and in the process expanded our understanding of the psychophysical basis of perimetry.

Important Physical Factors in Perimetry

The visibility of a light stimulus against a dimmer homogeneous background, the differential light sensitivity, is the basis for perimetric testing. In most perimeters the stimulus is projected upon, and hence added to, the brightness of the background illumination. Under light-adapted photopic conditions, the ratio of stimulus increment to background is a constant (Weber-Fechner law). However, as the background illumination becomes dimmer, and adaptation becomes mesopic or even scotopic, the constant no longer holds, and the relationship becomes nonlinear. Perimeters with dimmer background levels may begin to test in this nonlinear range if pupil size becomes smaller than 3 or 4 mm, or if significant lens opacity is present.

We can characterize the stimulus and background in a number of ways, but the commonest is in absolute units of luminance, such as apostilbs(asb), or relative units, such as log units or decibels (dB). Although absolute units may be easier to understand, and should be easier to standardize among different perimeters, differences in manufacture involving the stimulus light source, reflectance of the bowl surface, and other factors make standardization very difficult. Moreover, the human visual system responds more or less on a logarithmic scale to light intensity, so that the perceived change from 10 asb to 100 asb is roughly the same as that from 100 asb to 1,000 asb. Consequently, most automated perimeters have adopted the logarithmic, or decibel, scale to describe stimulus intensity, which varies throughout the test, but apostilbs to describe background intensity, which is stable throughout the test.

Every perimeter has a light source that determines its maximum stimulus intensity. In the decibel scale, this maximum intensity is assigned the value of 0 dB. Dimmer stimuli are expressed as the number of decibels less than the brightest possible stimulus. The higher the number, the dimmer the stimulus. Ten decibels is equivalent to one log unit. Thus, if the brightest possible stimulus is 10,000 asb and the chosen stimulus is 1,000 asb, the decibel number is 10. If the chosen stimulus is 100 asb, the decibel number is 20, and so forth. Observe that since higher numbers in decibels refer to dimmer stimuli, when printed on a visual field chart, a higher number means a greater retinal sensitivity.

The difference between the maximum stimulus brightness and the background level determines the dynamic range of a perimeter. If the maximum stimulus is relatively dim, say 1,000 asb as in the Octopus perimeters, then the background must be dimmer than the usual standard 31.5 asb in order to preserve a good dynamic range. As noted above, the Octopus 4 asb background level is still within the linear response curve of the retina, as long as small pupils or media opacities do not interfere. Maximum stimulus levels brighter than 10,000 asb produce light scattering beyond the borders of the stimulus, stimulating retina outside the test spot, and are therefore not practical. Dimmer background levels also show a less pronounced peak of foveal sensitivity relative to the surrounding areas of the field. Thus, visual field charts from perimeters with different background and stimulus characteristics do not have a predictable relationship to one another across the field.

Test object size is an important variable in perimetry. As Goldmann recognized long ago, spatial summation produces a certain interchangeability between test object size and brightness, a phenomenon that was exploited in the Goldmann perimeter. Most projection perimeters have chosen a Goldmann size III (4 mm^2) target for routine use because the effects of blur are less noticeable than with smaller test objects. Nonetheless, the importance of focusing the stimulus on the retina cannot be overemphasized. Corrective lenses appropriate for the patient's refraction and the distance of the perimeter bowl must be supplied for testing within the central 30 ° of field lest artifactual scotomas be introduced. Obviously the lens must be adjusted so that the rim does not interfere and must be removed for peripheral testing.

The length of time a stimulus is illuminated is also an important variable. Temporal summation occurs with presentations up to 0.5 seconds in clinical perimetry. Nonetheless, long presentation times encourage unstable fixation, so most perimeters use 0.1 or 0.2 seconds as a compromise.

Colored stimuli introduce a new set of variables. The level of dark adaptation is even more important than in white-light perimetry. The patient must also decide whether to respond when he first perceives the stimulus or whether to wait until it becomes the appropriate test color. Despite these concerns, further research in color perimetry continues because of a possible differential effect of certain diseases on the different chromatic systems. For example, the ganglion cell axons from the blue-cone system may be more susceptible to glaucomatous damage and show early defects when white-light perimetry is normal.

The Uncertainty Principle in Perimetry

In biologic systems, repeated measurements with the same parameter are subject to variability. Recall the LD50 concept from toxicology, a dose level at which half of the animals receiving a substance die from its toxic effects. In perimetry, threshold is defined as the stimulus level that is seen 50% of the time. Stimuli brighter than threshold are seen more than half of the time, but not 100% of the time until the stimulus is quite a bit brighter than threshold. Similarly, stimuli dimmer than threshold may be seen some of the time, not reaching 0% until the stimulus is substantially dimmer than threshold. This uncertainty of seeing the stimulus, or probability of seeing it, can be expressed in a frequency of seeing curve (Fig. 7.8).

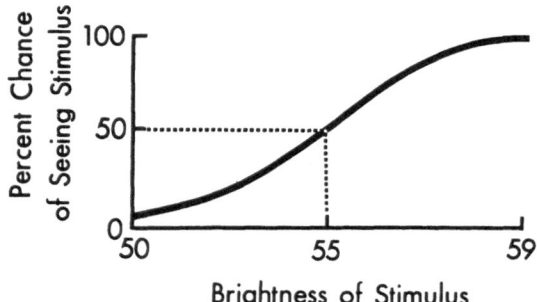

Figure 7.8. The uncertainty principle in perimetry. As a stimulus becomes brighter, the chance that it will be seen by the patient increases. The 50% level is called the threshold. In this example a stimulus of brightness 55 is seen half the time and not seen half the time. Brightness 55 thus represents the threshold for that point in this patient. However, in attempting to measure threshold, a stimulus of 50 will be seen 5% of the time and a stimulus of 58 will be missed 5% of the time. Multiple trials could establish a mean threshold, but time expenditure would be excessive if we tested many points.

Thus, the threshold as we measure it between seeing and nonseeing is not an absolute value, but instead is a border zone. The actual threshold, determined by taking the mean of multiple measurements, lies at the middle of the border zone. In fact, the threshold value we accept is always an estimate of the true threshold. The degree to which the estimate approximates the true threshold is dependent on the method we use to measure it and the number of times we measure it.

Threshold estimates are the numbers, expressed in decibels, with which we are familiar in charts of threshold static perimeters. However, the uncertainty of measuring threshold plays a role in kinetic and suprathreshold static perimetry as well. As we bring a kinetic stimulus centrally from the nonseeing periphery, the chances of seeing it gradually increase as we cross the border zone of threshold. On the basis of chance alone, a patient may see the stimulus at different eccentricities on multiple presentations. In suprathreshold static perimetry, we choose stimuli that are just above threshold. If they are too close, however, a certain number of presentations will be missed simply because the probability of a miss at one point is cumulated over the many points tested. Knowledge of that uncertainty has caused most suprathreshold testing programs to record misses only when the test spot has been missed twice. Even so, a certain percentage of test locations will be missed on the basis of chance alone.

In threshold static perimetry, if a few test locations are measured multiple times, or if all test locations are measured twice, a statistical measure of the uncertainty or variance can be calculated.

The slope of the frequency of seeing curve is fortunately quite steep in the majority of normal individuals. As the curve flattens in states of lowered alertness or in pathologic areas of the visual field, the uncertainty is magnified. For the clinician, the uncertainty of the visual field measurements represents a major source of frustration. There is a temptation to introduce shortcuts in the testing process on the grounds that field testing is inexact, at best. Such shortcuts usually result in an increased uncertainty to the point that the field data become uninterpretable.

Strategies for Determining Threshold

It is obviously impossible to measure threshold many times at each tested point, for we would use up our testing time before we gained much spatial information about the visual field. Consequently, it is necessary to develop strategies for estimating the threshold in a reasonably short time, accepting the fact that the threshold determination may not be very accurate.

In manual threshold static perimetry, the "ascending method of limits" was commonly used, in which threshold was approached from the nonseeing side in small steps until the first stimulus was seen -- and that was recorded as threshold. In most automated perimeters, an up-down staircase method is employed since the computer can test the points randomly and the patient cannot focus attention on a point at which he or she saw the stimulus. In this method, if the first point is seen, the stimulus is made dimmer in large steps until missed, then brighter again in small steps until seen. Conversely, if the first point is missed, the stimulus is made brighter in large steps until seen, then dimmer again in small steps until missed. Thus, the threshold is crossed twice in most bracketing strategies, although some algorithms cross threshold three or even more, at the expense of increased test time.

If the initial presentation is close to threshold, fewer steps will be required to cross threshold, and test time will be saved. Some bracketing strategies utilize normative data stored in the computer to determine the strength of the initial stimulus at each point. Others may use threshold data determined on the initial four "primary" points to determine the start levels for subsequent points. In such a case, threshold at the primary points is usually determined twice to minimize the effect of spurious values. Or, if the patient has previously undergone threshold perimetry, the previous threshold determinations may be used ("full from prior data" strategy).

Patterns of Test Points

It is theoretically impossible to map the entire visual field since regardless of how many test points were selected, there would still be room between them for more points. Obviously, we would like to retain sufficient density of test point locations to detect scotomas of the size of the physiologic blind spot, for instance. The time constraints of threshold static perimetry have forced us to accept point densities that are marginal in terms of that criterion. A standard grid of 76 equally spaced points in a rectangular array within the central 30° has a point situated every 6° in horizontal and vertical directions, and every 9° diagonally. It is no wonder that the physiologic blind spot is not discovered on a significant number of Humphrey 30-2 or Octopus 32 fields. Other than the advantage of predictable point density, and ease of grey scale interpolation, there is no reason to test the field using a rectangular grid of points. Field defects do not affect all areas of the central field with equal frequency, and point arrays might be designed in the future with that in mind.

If the point density in threshold static testing of the central field is marginal, it is even less so peripherally. Time constraints limit testing to the area between 30° and 60° of eccentricity, and with point spacings of 12° (17° diagonally). Variability of threshold determinations in the midperiphery of the field is also quite high. Therefore, routine threshold testing of the field beyond 30° may not be a worthwhile use of test time.

Denser point arrays can be designed for suprathreshold testing because each point is tested only once (twice for missed points). They also can be arranged in areas where field defects are most likely to be encountered in various disease states. The perimetrist can then make a program selection based on the expected pathology. The objective of such testing is screening for defects; once they are found, more quantitative methods such as threshold static testing may still need to be applied to use as a baseline against which to evaluate future change.

Program selection for quantitative testing is generally easier, since two constraints limit the choices. First, if a patient is to be evaluated for change over time, the field test should be the same on each test occasion. As more and more patients are tested with a standard program, it becomes more difficult to convert to a different standard. Second, if the field is to be compared statistically to a normal database, the test conditions must be the same as used on the normal population. Collection of such normative data is extremely time consuming and costly, and this has been accomplished for only a few quantitative programs on the Octopus and Humphrey perimeters. From a practical point of view, Programs 31, 32, and G1 on the Octopus 201 perimeter and programs 30-1 and 30-2 or 24-1 and 24-2 on the Humphrey perimeter are the current workhorses for the majority of patient testing. The special programs that test only the central 10°, the midperiphery, a selected area within the field, a meridian, or user-defined programs are used for more specialized purposes or not at all.

Kinetic perimetry seems best suited for testing in the periphery of the field, but it is not known whether such testing improves the detection rate of field defects over central threshold static testing alone. Some automated perimeters have the capability for peripheral kinetic testing, though such strategies have not yet been validated.

Important Variables to Control in Perimetry

Background and stimulus luminances are automatically adjusted to standard values by most computerized perimeters, but it is wise to have a service technician recalibrate the instrument during routine maintenance. On manual perimeters and on tangent screens, the task of calibration is left to the perimetrist; if not done regularly, results from serial fields may not be comparable. Similarly, stimulus presentation durations and interstimulus intervals are internally adjusted on automated units, but perimetrists need to be consistent in their technique in manual perimetry.

The stimulus must be focused on the retina. Provision of corrective lenses for testing beyond 30° is not practical, but centrally it is essential. Failure to provide appropriate lens correction is the commonest error in clinical perimetry. Costs of the error include the appearance of refractive scotomas and an apparent reduction in light sensitivity (Heuer et al, 1987). Starting with the patient's distance refraction, an age-appropriate additional correction for the distance from the eye to the perimeter bowl is factored into the corrective lens(es) used during testing. Most of the time, testing may be done using the same corrective lens(es) employed during the patient's previous visual field, but care should be taken that the patient has not developed a refractive change, such as lenticular myopia, in the interim. Pupil size must also be larger than 2.5 mm; if it is not, the pupil should be dilated prior to perimetry.

Patients are, in a sense, the largest uncontrolled variable in perimetry. Individual variations in levels of cooperation and understanding are enormous, yet these can be minimized through proper instruction and ongoing monitoring. The patient must be as comfortable as possible during the test. The chair and headrest adjustments take some time but pay dividends in result reliability. Patients need to be told what is expected of them. For example, the response button should be pushed only when they are reasonably sure the stimulus has appeared. They do not need to respond during the time the stimulus is actually illuminated. Most of the stimuli are quite dim, and sometimes the machine makes noises as though a stimulus is being shown, but none appears. Patients need human feedback during the test, including encouragement that they are doing well, admonishment to look at the center, instructions appropriate to correct a high false-positive or negative rate, and position adjustments. Such adjustments are critical to avoid "fixation losses" caused by movement of the physiologic blind spot away from its original location (this is usually due to a sideways head tilt) and to avoid trial lens rim artifact from backward tilt of the head away from the forehead rest.

There is a definite learning effect in automated perimetry. For the average patient, this is a significant variable only for the first automated field. It is therefore advisable to perform an introductory field before the actual scheduled first examination. Otherwise the results obtained may not be useful in comparing with subsequent fields, in which the performance level has improved.

Some variables cannot be controlled at all. Patients may feel poorly, be distracted by stressful events, or feel anxious about the test to the detriment of their performance. Sometimes it is necessary simply to reschedule the examination at a more propitious time.

Data Representation and Pitfalls -- Sources of Artifact

Results from a kinetic field are plotted by connecting the stimulus response points, forming the familiar isopter map. Printouts from static automated perimeters are less familiar to practitioners. Suprathreshold test results are usually presented as maps, with missed stimulus locations appearing as dark dots or squares and seen locations as fainter symbols. To interpret these patterns it is necessary to know the test strategy used. It can usually be found somewhere on the printout.

Data from static threshold perimetry appear as threshold numbers on a visual field map. Careful scrutiny of such printouts is necessary to extract the important information. Even so, it is difficult to identify subtle areas of depression or categorize scotoma shape from numeric printouts.

Consequently, gray scale representations have become popular. Each range of threshold values is assigned a shade of gray (density of dots in the dot-matrix array) and areas between the measured points are arithmetically interpolated. When using gray scale displays, it is important to remember that the interpolations may be misleading. In addition, the printer ribbon may be of different age on consecutive tests, leading to a "darker" or "lighter" impression of the whole field. Automated visual fields should be interpreted by analysis of the numerical data (with statistical analysis if available). The gray scale alone should not be used as the sole basis for clinical decisions.

Another pitfall can result from so-called difference printouts. Some of these rely on normative data stored in the computer memory; the patient's thresholds are subtracted from the normal thresholds and the differences are recorded on the printout. Since the normal data are age-corrected, the patient's birth date must have been correctly entered, or the "differences" may be artifactual. Another type of difference printout subtracts the actual measured thresholds from the expected thresholds based on extrapolation from the first several points tested. If this type of difference printout is resident in the original software, and an upgrade is purchased that uses the difference based on normative data, the difference printouts will appear radically different on serial fields spanning the date of the software change.

Patient positioning errors are a frequent source of artifact. An overhanging brow, drooping upper lid, large nose, or trial lens placed too far from the eye will each produce focal depressions in the periphery. A patient may gradually change position during testing, introducing artifacts that were absent initially.

The peripheral ring of points in a central 30° field have the lowest sensitivity, the highest variability, and the greatest range of normality. Often, they may indicate an artifactual defect. However, it is unwise to omit the peripheral points from testing because they may be helpful in confirming a defect that extends more centrally. As mentioned in the preceding section, failure to provide the appropriate corrective lens(es) for testing within the central 30° can easily produce artifactual scotomas which mimic bona fide disease.

Artifacts can also be produced by certain types of inappropriate patient behavior. Trigger-happy patients who respond to the noises made by the perimeter or other nonvisual cues may achieve visual thresholds well out of the physiologic range (40-60 dB). In addition, there will be a high false-positive rate caused by responses to sham stimuli. If patient instruction to lower the false-positive rate is not effective, such fields should probably be considered invalid, since significant scotomas may be missed entirely. Patients with high false-negative rates are usually inattentive (but not always continuously so) and need to be reminded to concentrate on the task. If lower false-negative rates cannot be achieved, the field should be regarded with suspicion, especially as regards general or focal depression, but may still contain useful information. It is also wise to remember that some patients with pathologic fields may score high false-negative rates in spite of adequate cooperation (Heijl et al, 1987b). In perimeters using periodic stimulus presentations within the physiologic blind spot as a measure of fixation accuracy, a high fixation loss rate lends less credence to the validity of the field. However, drift in patient position, especially lateral head tilt, may cause a relocation of the blind spot to a position away from the blind spot check location, causing an artifactually high fixation loss rate.

Data Analysis -- Pattern vs. Statistical

The human brain is highly organized to recognize patterns. Facial recognition is a nearly instantaneous process for most people, yet computers are virtually unable to match a facial image acquired under different conditions to the one in resident memory. Much of visual field interpretation is an exercise in pattern recognition and is performed very well by people. Computers can, however, provide assistance to this process through application of statistical manipulations to the data. In so doing, the probabilistic nature of the visual field data is considered, and the power of the ultimate interpretation is increased. It is probably a misconception that the interpretive process will ever be performed solely by the computer because of the importance of pattern recognition in the process.

A variety of statistical packages for analysis of visual field data have appeared and will continue to be refined. Both the Humphrey and Octopus perimeters can calculate four visual field indices from the data in a standard central test. Mean defect or mean deviation (MD) is the depression of sensitivity from age-corrected normal values averaged across all tested points. Short-term fluctuation (SF) is the intratest variability calculated from selected points in the field which were tested twice. It has two components, which cannot as yet be separated. Short-term fluctuation may be elevated because the patient is inattentive or not cooperating consistently, or because the field is abnormal, for pathologic points show increased fluctuation (Flammer et al, 1984). Loss variance (LV) or pattern standard deviation (PSD) is a measure of the unevenness of the field - that is, are some of the points contributing most of the abnormality. Because patients with a high SF will also score high LV or PSD because of the high variability, one can apply a correction factor based on SF, yielding an index known as corrected loss variance (CLV) or corrected pattern standard deviation (CPSD). Each of the indices is helpful in identifying possible abnormalities that may be searched for on the numeric or gray scale printouts for confirmation.

The Humphrey perimeter statistical package (Statpak) (Heijl et al, 1987a) has another aid to identify abnormalities in single field examinations. From an age-corrected normal database, the chance that a measured threshold is normal can be displayed. The probability that individual points are not normal can be easily identified, even though they may not be obvious on the standard printouts. In viewing such probability maps, it is useful to remember that at the 5% probability level, in a 76-point field, 4 points in a truly normal field will be flagged on the basis of chance alone. At the 2% level, 2 points; at the 1% level, 1 point; and at the 0.5% level, 1 point in a pair of fields. Clustering of points that are significantly different from normal is a more troublesome sign than isolated abnormal points.

Finally, in interpreting probability maps or any statistical data that rely on a normal database, one must remember the assumption that the patient is behaving as the normals of his age did. If his performance is substandard on the reliability indices, or even on other criteria that are not measured by the perimeter, the probability statements are invalid.

A more complex task is the identification of change in serial visual fields. Printing the fields sequentially on a single piece of paper is useful in subjective analysis, but there is evidence that no consistent conclusions are drawn by expert observers asked to interpret a series of fields from the same patient (Werner et al, 1988). Evidently, criteria for clinically significant change are not agreed upon by those interpreting visual fields.

Much hope was therefore vested in statistical means of comparing consecutive fields for progression, stability, or improvement. One approach is to graph the visual field indices over time and apply t-tests to paired mean values. Another is a regression analysis to determine if significant change has occurred. When Werner applied six different statistical techniques to series of fields from the same patients, no consistent conclusions could be drawn about whether change had occurred (Werner et al, 1988). From a clinical perspective, the problem of longitudinal analysis is further complicated by the effects of treatment change(s) applied during the time of observation, which distort the natural history of the disease. From a statistical perspective, the assumption that the visual field data are independent observations that are normally distributed is probably incorrect (Heijl, 1987; Heijl et al, 1987c), thus invalidating conclusions drawn by most analyses that have been applied to date. On the other hand, the application of statistics to visual field data is in its infancy, and better methods of analysis are to be expected in the future.

Recent Studies by Investigator and Others

Validation of Perimeters

As Keltner (1981) has pointed out, clinical use of a perimeter and software that have not been validated against a previously established standard is risky. Small differences in manufacture or in the testing algorithms may have substantial effect on the test results. Fortunately, many automated perimeters that were never validated have disappeared from the marketplace. Among currently available perimeters, the Fieldmaster 101PR (Johnson and Keltner, 1980) and 200 (Mills, 1984b), Dicon 2000 (Mills, 1984b), Octopus 201 (Kriegelstein et al, 1981), Competer (Heijl, 1976), and Humphrey (Mills et al, 1986; (Trope and Britton, 1987) have good validation studies published in the literature.

Effectiveness of Interactive Software

In suprathreshold screening perimetry, it is difficult to achieve sensitivity levels (percent of truly abnormal fields identified as such on screening) in excess of 90% while maintaining an acceptable specificity level (percent of normal fields identified as such on screening). A variety of enhancements to simple screening algorithms have been tested to date. On the Dicon perimeter, programs that tested the depth of scotomas identified in screening and that tried to fit the stimulus intensity very close to the expected threshold of that patient were not successful in improving sensitivity, but actually caused a deterioration in specificity (Mills, 1985a). On the Humphrey perimeter, a program that surrounded each missed point with a cluster of additional test points to improve spatial resolution did not result in a better sensitivity/specificity mix (Asman et al, 1989). One of the problems seems to be that some visual fields of normal individuals contain areas of slightly depressed sensitivity that are detected as abnormal by programs sensitive enough to detect most true pathology (Asman et al, 1989; Heijl and Asman, 1989).

Usefulness of Peripheral vs. Central Field Testing

In the stampede to automated perimetry, peripheral field testing has fallen into disuse. The reason is that threshold testing takes a lot of time, and threshold values are more variable in the periphery. Test time seems more parsimoniously spent centrally. But in so doing, there is concern that significant field defects might be missed or incorrect visual field diagnoses assigned (Wirtschafter, 1987).

In suprathreshold screening perimetry, the peripheral field data did not add appreciably to the detection of abnormality, but it did increase the confidence level of the diagnostic impression based on the central field alone (Mills, 1985b).

When abnormalities appear on a central 30° static threshold test, confirmation of the diagnostic impression is often desirable. Three options for confirmation include a repetition of the 30° central threshold test, a peripheral screening test, or peripheral quantitative testing. A study of the first two options in 92 patients concluded that for nasal depression, focal peripheral depressions, and hemianopias, a peripheral screening test was a better option, but for all other types of defect on the initial central test, a repetition of central testing was advisable (Zamber and Mills, 1989). Quantitative testing of the peripheral nasal field has been shown to provide information in glaucoma detection additional to that provided by central testing (Seamone et al, 1989). Automated kinetic perimetry to provide peripheral isopters in addition to central threshold static data has produced promising early results (Johnson et al, 1987; Stewart et al, 1988). Unfortunately, at this time no commercially available automated perimeter provides a kinetic capability.

Future of the Test

Statistical Advances in Light-Sense Perimetry

Correlations of the existing visual field indices (MD, SF, LV, or PSD, and CLV or CPSD) with contrast sensitivity (Zulauf and Flammer, 1989) and with neuroretinal rim area (Wijsman et al, 1989) have recently appeared. As further clinical correlations are generated, the diagnostic usefulness of the indices will doubtless improve. For example, it would be particularly useful to be able to separate the variance due to personal factors (such as attentiveness) from the remainder of SF due to pathologic changes in the visual field. Additional global visual field indices may prove to be of value, particularly those that are spatially sensitive such as spatial correlation (Bebie, 1985) and cluster analysis (Chauhan et al, 1989), but they will require rigorous clinical validation. The application of artificial intelligence to automated perimetry (Krakau, 1987) also holds considerable promise.

In automated perimetry, SF is estimated using double determinations of selected points in the field, requiring additional test time. Recent studies have indicated that SF can be estimated mathematically by trend surface analysis of a visual field data grid without any double determinations (Mills et al, 1987; Schulzer et al, 1989), thus saving considerable test time.

A major challenge for the future of statistical analysis in perimetry is the detection of significant change over time. The intratest variability (SF) and intratest variability (long-term fluctuation) is sufficiently large in most patients that only a relatively large incremental change can reach statistical significance (Katz and Sommer, 1987). Thus, there are only a finite number of steps between normal vision and blindness that can be statistically identified. As investigation proceeds, we may be unpleasantly surprised by how few steps there are. That is not to say that light-sense perimetry will have less clinical value, but only that we will have a more realistic view of its capabilities.

Blue/Yellow Testing

Because patients with ocular hypertension and glaucoma are known to have a high prevalence of defective blue/yellow discrimination on foveal color testing, it is logical to attempt visual field testing of the blue-cone system. To isolate the blue cones, it is necessary to have a very bright yellow background or other color receptors will respond to the blue target. Very early results have indicated no preferential loss in the blue-yellow system in early glaucoma (Johnson et al, 1989) and no clinically useful improved ability to detect defects not found in conventional white-light perimetry (Hart, 1989). Research in perimetry to isolate a differential effect of glaucoma on color or other psychophysical function will continue and may yet result in a useful clinical test.

"Ring" Perimetry

It has long been recognized that traditional light-sense perimetry does not maximally stimulate the receptive field properties of human ganglion cells. The problem with more complicated targets, such as visual acuity optotypes or sinusoidal gratings, in the peripheral field is that there are two visual thresholds. The first threshold is recognition (something there) and the second is resolution (letter "E" or orientation of the grating).

The confusion in the response criterion increases variability of response and reduces clinical usefulness.

Stimuli that have nearly equivalent detection and resolution thresholds, known as vanishing or high-pass resolution targets, circumvent this problem. (Howland et al, 1978). Frisén (1987) has applied the technique to perimetry using ring-shaped targets presented on a video screen. The average luminance of the target is identical to the background. The ring itself is lighter than the background and is surrounded by concentric borders that are darker than the background. The width of the ring and the black borders are 1/5 and 1/20 of the ring diameter, respectively. The size of the ring is varied during the examination

Peripheral sensitivity to these targets can be expressed as a type of acuity, the minimum angle of resolution (MAR). Interestingly, the relationship in normals between MAR with the ring test and reported density of human ganglion cells is linear. With increasing eccentricity, as acuity decreases, so does the density of ganglion cells (Frisén, 1987).

Early results indicate the "ring test" correlates well with conventional perimetry in established glaucoma (Dannheim et al, 1989a), demyelinating optic neuropathy (Cox and Douglas, 1989), and chiasmal disease (Dannheim et al, 1989b). There is some indication that ocular hypertensives, patients with early glaucoma (Wanger and Persson, 1987), and patients with subclinical optic neuropathy (Cox and Douglas, 1989) may show more defects on the "ring test" than on conventional perimetry. However, as with any new tests that appear to be more sensitive than conventional tests, we must discover during clinical validation whether the "ring test" has an acceptable false-alarm rate among truly normal individuals.

As currently configured, the "ring test" has several advantages in difficult testing situations:

1. Standard test time is about 5 minutes per eye. A standard examination on most light-sense automated perimeters takes at least twice as long.

2. The test has ongoing patient feedback. After the patient responds, a black square target appears where the test target had been projected. The patient becomes more involved in the testing.

3. The computer and test monitor are portable and can be set up at the bedside.

Currently the "ring test" is limited to testing within the central visual field because of the restrictions of the video monitor and has a limited dynamic range. With improvements in liquid crystal display technology, it is conceivable that ring-shaped or other stimuli could be presented on a hemispheric surface like a perimeter bowl and, in addition, boost the dynamic range of the instrument.

Testing Methods Directed to Receptive Field Properties

Basic research into the mechanisms of damage from glaucoma and the morphology, distribution, and properties of primate ganglion cells may suggest other methods of testing to identify early damage to one or more functional channels in glaucoma and other diseases. As such tests are developed, the confounding variable of the human patient must always be considered. No matter how refined we become in automated perimetry, until we are able to eliminate the patient-response button, the physician's clinical judgment will always be required.

Summary

Automated perimetry has, within only a few years, become the dominant force in perimetry in many parts of the world. This revolution has been all the more remarkable because it has entailed a change from the standard kinetic method of visual field exploration to static threshold perimetry, a type of testing previously seldom practiced outside research institutions. As it turns out, static threshold perimetry offers several advantages over kinetic testing. Most important among them are an increased sensitivity in detecting early defects, a suitability for statistical analysis of the data, and a relative ease of developing test logic for automation. Static stimuli of suprathreshold intensity may also be applied to screening applications, most effectively when the intensity of the stimulus is closely related to the expected threshold (threshold-related suprathreshold static testing).

Because in perimetry we are attempting to measure a patient's threshold between seeing and nonseeing, there is an inherent variability in the response. This fluctuation increases in poorly cooperative patients and in disease, and it must be taken into account when deciding whether a field is abnormal, or whether a field has changed between two examinations.

Interpretation of automated visual fields is subject to a variety of pitfalls related to the peculiarities of data display, especially gray scale and "difference" printouts. Human skills at recognizing patterns of visual field defect can be helped by statistical analysis of the data performed by the computer. Identification of abnormal single visual fields is assisted by the so-called visual field indices and by probability maps indicating the likelihood that a tested point is normal. A more complicated task is the identification of significant change over time. At present, no statistical method is available to do that reliably.

In the future, statistical analysis of visual field data will improve. Other methods of perimetry involving more complicated targets than white circles of light may help to improve sensitivity in detecting early disease. However, such improved sensitivity may be achieved only at the expense of a a decreased specificity (high false-alarm rate in normals). Only further research will provide the answer. In the meantime, the automation of perimetry has at least made clinical visual field testing easier to do, thus leading to significant improvement in our ability to care for patients.

References

Asman P, Britt JM, Mills RP, Heijl A. Evaluation of adaptive spatial enhancement in suprathreshold visual field screening. Ophthalmology 1988;95:1656-62.

Bebie H. Computerized techniques of visual field analysis. In Drance SM , Anderson DR (eds) Automatic perimetry in glaucoma - a practical guide. Orlando: Grune and Stratton: 1985;pp. 147-60.

Chauhan BC, Henson DB, Hobley AJ. Cluster analysis in visual field quantification. In Heijl A (ed) Proceedings of the eighth international visual field symposium. Amsterdam: Kugler: 1989; in press.

Cox TA, Douglas GR. High-pass resolution perimetry in multiple sclerosis. In Heijl A (ed) Proceedings of the eighth international visual field symposium. Amsterdam: Kugler: 1989; in press.

Dannheim F, Abramo F, Verlohr D. Comparison of automated conventional and spatial resolution perimetry in glaucoma. In Heijl A (ed) Proceedings of the eighth international visual field symposium. Amsterdam: Kugler: 1989a; in press.

Dannheim F, Roggenbuck C. Comparison of automated conventional and spatial resolution perimetry in chiasmal lesions. In Heijl A (ed) Proceedings of the eighth international visual field symposium. Amsterdam: Kugler: 1989b; in press.

Fankhauser F, Koch P, Roulier A. On automation of perimetry. Albrecht Von Graefes Arch Klin Exp Ophthalmol 1972;184:126-50.

Ferree CE, Rand G, Sloan LL. Selected cases showing the advantages of a combined tangent screen and perimeter. Arch Ophthalmol 1933;10:166-84.

Flammer J, Drance SM, Fankhauser F, Augustiny L. Differential light threshold in automated static perimetry - factors influencing short-term fluctuation. Arch Ophthalmol 1984;102:876-9.

Frisén L. High-pass resolution targets in peripheral vision. Ophthalmology 1987;94:1104-8.

Harms H, Aulhorn E. Vergleichende untersuchungen uber den wert der quantitativen perimetrie, skiaskotometrie und verschmelzungsfrequenz fur die erkennjng beginnender gesichtsfeldstorungen beim glaukom. Doc Ophthalmol 1959;13:303-32.

Hart WM. Blue/yellow color contrast perimetry compared to conventional kinetic perimetry in patients with established glaucomatous visual field defects. In Heijl A (ed) Proceedings of the eighth international visual field symposium. Amsterdam: Kugler: 1989; in press.

Heijl A, Krakau CET. An automatic perimeter for glaucoma visual field screening and control. Albrecht Von Graefes Arch Klin Exp Ophthalmol 1975;197:13-23.

Heijl A. Automatic perimetry in glaucoma visual field screening. Albrecht Von Graefes Arch Klin Exp Ophthalmol 1976;200:21-37.

Heijl A. The implications of the results of computerized perimetry in normals for the statistical evaluation of glaucomatous visual fields. In Krieglstein GK (ed) Glaucoma Update III. Berlin: Springer-Verlag: 1987;pp. 115-22.

Heijl A, Lindgren G, Olsson J. A package for the statistical analysis of visual fields. Doc Ophthalmol Proc Ser 1987a;49:153-68.

Heijl A, Lindgren G, Olsson J. Reliability parameters in computerized perimetry. Doc Ophthalmol Proc Ser 1987b;49:593-600.

Heijl A, Lindgren G, Olsson J. Normal variability of static perimetric threshold values across the central visual field. Doc Ophthalmol Proc Ser 1987c;105:1544-9.

Heijl A, Asman P. Clustering of depressed points in the normal visual field. In Heijl A (ed) Proceedings of the eighth international visual field symposium. Amsterdam: Kugler: 1989; in press.

Heuer DK, Anderson DR, Feuer WJ, Gressel MG. The influence of refraction accuracy on automated perimetric threshold measurements. Ophthalmology 1987;94:1550-3.

Howland B, Ginsburg A, Compbell F. High-pass spatial frequency letters as clinical optotypes. Vis Res 1978;18:1063-6.

Johnson CA, Keltner JL. Comparative evaluation of the Autofield-I, CFA-110, and Fieldmaster 101 PR automated perimeters. Ophthalmology 1980;87:777-84.

Johnson CA, Keltner JL, Lewis RA. Automated kinetic perimetry. an efficient method of evaluating peripheral visual field loss. Appl Opt 1987;26:1409-14.

Johnson CA, Adams AJ, Lewis, RA. Automated perimetry of blue-sensitive mechanisms in ocular hypertension and early glaucoma. In Heijl A (ed) Proceedings of the eighth international visual field symposium. Amsterdam: Kugler: 1989; in press.

Katz J, Sommer A. A longitudinal study of the age-adjusted variability of automated visual fields. Arch Ophthalmol 1987;105:1083-86.

Keltner JL. Automated perimetry - a consumer's guide. Ann Ophthalmol 1981;pp. 275-9.

Krakau CET. Artificial intelligence in computerized perimetry. Doc Ophthalmol Proc Ser 1987;49:169-74.

Kriegelstein GK, Schrems W, Gramer E, Leydhecker W. Detectability of early glaucomatous field defects - a controlled comparison of Goldmann versus Octopus perimetry. Doc Ophthalmol Proc Ser 1981;26:19-24.

Mills RP. Automated perimetry, part I. Am Intraoc Implant Soc J 1984a;10:347-53.

Mills RP. A comparison of Goldmann, Fieldmaster 200, and Dicon AP2000 perimeters used in a screening mode. Ophthalmology 1984b;91:347-54.

Mills RP. Evaluation of diagnostic capabilities of interactive test strategies in automated perimetry. Ophthalmology 1985a;92:1181-6.

Mills RP. Usefulness of peripheral testing in automated screening perimetry. Doc Ophthalmol Proc Ser 1985b;42:207-11.

Mills RP, Hopp RH, Drance SM. Comparison of quantitative testing with the Octopus, Humphrey, and Tubingen perimeters. Am J Ophthalmol 1986;12:496-504.

Mills RP, Schulzer M, Hopp RH, Drance SM. Estimates of variance in visual field data. Doc Ophthalmol Proc Ser 1987;49:93-101.

Rock WJ, Drance SM, Morgan RW. A modification of the Armaly visual field screening technique for glaucoma. Can J Ophthalmol 1971;6:283-92.

Schulzer M, Mills RP, Hopp RH, Drance SM. Variance estimates from threshold grid patterns. In Heijl A (ed) Proceedings of the eighth international visual field symposium. Amsterdam: Kugler: 1989; in press.

Seamone C, LeBlanc RP, Mann C, Rubillowicz M, Orr A. The value of indices in the central and peripheral visual field in the detection of glaucoma. In Heijl A (ed) Proceedings of the eighth international visual field symposium. Amsterdam: Kugler: 1989; in press.

Stewart WC, Shields MB, Ollie AR. Peripheral visual field testing by automated kinetic perimetry in glaucoma. Arch Ophthalmol 1988;106:202-6.

Traquair HM. Introduction to Clinical Perimetry. London. Kimpton:1927.

Trope GE, Britton R. A comparison of Goldmann and Humphrey automated perimetry in patients with glaucoma. Br J Ophthalmol 1987;71:489-93.

Wanger P, Persson HE. Pattern-reversal electroretinograms and high-pass resolution perimetry in suspected or early glaucoma. Ophthalmology 1987;94:1098-1103.

Werner EB, Bishop KI, Koelle J, et al. A comparison of experienced clinical observes and statistical tests in detecting progressive visual field loss in glaucoma using automated perimetry. Arch Ophthalmol 1988;106:619-23.

Wijsman K, Schulzer M, Drance SM, Douglas GR. The correlation between neuroretinal rim and visual field indices. In Heijl A (ed) Proceedings of the eighth international visual field symposium. Amsterdam: Kugler: 1989; in press.

Wirtschafter JD. Examination of the peripheral visual field - obligatory, helpful, or a waste of resources. Arch Ophthalmol 1987;105:761-2.

Zamber R, Mills RP. Peripheral vs. central confirmatory testing. In Heijl A (ed) Proceedings of the eighth international visual field symposium. Amsterdam: Kugler: 1989; in press.

Zulauf M, Flammer J. Visual field indices and their correlation with contrast sensitivity in glaucoma--preliminary results. In Heijl A (ed) Proceedings of the eighth international visual field symposium. Amsterdam: Kugler: 1989; in press.

Index